RESTORING YOUR LIFE ENERGY

Also by Master Waysun Liao

Chi
The Essence of T'ai Chi
T'ai Chi Classics

—RESTORING YOUR— LIFE ENERGY

Simple Chi Gung Practices to Reduce Stress and Enhance Well-Being

Master Waysun Liao

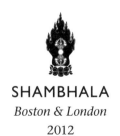

SHAMBHALA

Boston & London

2012

Shambhala Publications, Inc.
Horticultural Hall
300 Massachusetts Avenue
Boston, Massachusetts 02115
www.shambhala.com

9 8 7 6 5 4 3 2 1

First Edition
Printed in the United States of America

⊗ This edition is printed on acid-free paper that meets
the American National Standards Institute Z39.48 Standard.
♻ This book is printed on 30% postconsumer recycled paper.
For more information please visit www.shambhala.com.

Distributed in the United States by Random House, Inc.,
and in Canada by Random House of Canada Ltd

Designed by James D. Skatges

Library of Congress Cataloging-in-Publication Data

Liao, Waysun, 1948– -
Restoring your life energy: simple chi gung practices to reduce stress
and enhance well-being / Waysun Liao.—First Edition.
pages cm
Includes bibliographical references and index.
ISBN 978-1-59030-996-4 (pbk.)
1. Qi gong. 2. Exercise therapy. 3. Stress management. I. Title.
RA781.8.L54 2012
613.71489—dc23
2012005548

CONTENTS

RESTORING YOUR LIFE ENERGY

INTRODUCTION

In today's busy life, full of sorrow and exhilaration, demands and challenges, noise and toxins, information overload and nonstop activity, it's easy to feel drained, scattered, stressed, or run-down. Over time, the assault of modern living can even take its toll on our physical health and inner well-being. A quiet desire inside many people whispers, *How can I recharge myself? How can I feel as energetic, clear, and vibrant as I remember feeling in my youth?*

It's hard to find the real answers to those questions. One reason is because so many fake answers flash at us from every television, magazine, billboard, radio, and Internet ad. Since everyone is looking for more energy, more youth, and more vitality, businesses and advertisers parade out countless products and services claiming to deliver some sort of "recharging" power. How about an island vacation? Cosmetic surgery? A new sports car? Energy drinks? Maybe you just need a new prescription drug to make you feel more alive.

However, many people find that these answers don't deliver the real vitality and sense of aliveness they really seek—at least not over the long term. If such products did work, word would have leaked out to everyone else, and we'd all be vivacious, centered, healthy, and happy.

Do you know what that unfulfilled longing is? That push to find a way to recharge yourself? It is actually your life energy crying out for help!

We keep looking for modern-day answers to a long-standing dilemma: How can we restore our life energy? The irony is that we will most likely find the answer to that question in a centuries-old path hidden among the brambles of time.

That hidden path was trod by ancient pioneers we now call Taoists. Long ago, Taoists searched for answers to some of the same questions that overwhelm us today. Without television or self-help seminars, they were forced to practice deep meditation as a way to find those answers. Through that deep meditation, they gradually understood the secrets of life energy, or what they called *chi* (pronounced *chee*). They learned the secrets of chi directly from their own experience. They gained firsthand understanding by using themselves—their bodies, their minds, their breathing, their lifestyles—as objects of practice. Through trial and error over the centuries, they evolved the full range of Taoist knowledge: acupuncture, healing, herbal medicine, martial arts, spiritual reading, feng shui, chi gung, t'ai chi, Tao gung, and more.

Some of these ancient "internal energy" explorers went even deeper and discovered that within and underlying their chi was a spark of higher-level, more refined power. They called this even more rarefied form of original life energy *yuan chi*, or "one chi." They realized that this spark of energy held even greater potential for personal transformation than normal chi. By reaching it, they could go beyond simply feeling more energetic and enjoying better health. They sensed that this spark gave each person infinite potential.

When they realized that everyone has a bit of this yuan chi, they knew they had discovered a profound truth: human beings have a spark of what might be termed God right inside us. They called this spark of original energy deep within each person the *Te* (pronounced *day*). They came to understand that this Te served as each person's inner connection to the One Universal Energy. Through deeper meditation and lifetimes of practice, they came to experience their Te as a gateway they could use to travel back to God. Their word for the ever-present, all-intelligent, infinite power of God or Source is *Tao*.

Part of the practice they did to reach their Te was to clean and strengthen their life energy. They called this type of practice *chi gung,* which literally means "chi's work." They did chi gung so they could bring their life energy to its ultimate and purest state. That state of ultimate chi is *t'ai chi.* In fact, an advanced application of chi gung moving meditation is what we now know as t'ai chi practice. When the ancient practitioners reached the state of t'ai chi, they could use the energy to drill down inside themselves to their Te and connect to the Tao. They had a series of special meditation practices called *Tao gung,* literally "Tao's work," to reach this state.

Usually, the early Taoists practiced chi gung, t'ai chi, and Tao gung. They devoted their entire lives to accommodating their practice so they could make better progress. Only those with very strong, pure life energy—energy refined and trained through the three practices—could contact the internal Te and hope to reach their ultimate goal.

What was that goal? Originally, the Taoists sought to reach eternity. They wanted to fuse themselves to the Tao through their life energy so they could live forever. However, they did not want to live forever in this dimension. Their true goal was to find a way to travel through the gateway of Te inside and enter the eternal dimension. They believed this gateway could transport them beyond the restrictions of our own dimension—the realm of birth and death, space and time—and they would be able to immerse themselves in the highest dimension of original universal energy.

It was this goal that spurred the ancients onward in their meditation, their chi gung exercises, and their arts. The interesting thing is that we have records giving us good reason to believe that some of them made it! We have the memoirs, practice books, and temple legends of famous masters and highly accomplished Taoist saints called immortals. We also have hints in the historical records of miraculous transformations performed by a few of these masters and saints. Ancient government scrolls show that some of these accomplished monks appear to have reached considerable age, living 120, 136, and in some cases, more than 200 years, while still remaining active in the temple or even in public life.

Yet we can only piece together fragments of these old saints' lives. If you set out to find their true, effective chi gung practices and use them with the correct wisdom of those old masters' original teachings, you would most likely dig for years through dusty scrolls and arcane books that sometimes make no sense. Alternately, you could wander all over the world trying to find a real master who had achieved the state of t'ai chi or even experienced the Tao. That might take you many years, and you would undoubtedly encounter many exuberant and compelling teachers who could offer only partial truths. You'd have about as much luck finding an authentic and true master as you would looking for a real twenty dollar bill in a sea of expert counterfeits.

Because the old monks believed that mastery over chi might be dangerous in the wrong hands, the knowledge and practices they developed were kept within a very small and exclusive lineage. The teachings were usually passed down secretly from generation to generation within the confines of a temple or a reclusive mountain community far from regular society.

Over the centruies, some of this knowledge and select practices found their way into Taoist texts. However, we'd have to spend many years struggling to decode these texts in order to decipher what we'd need to know to restore our chi. This is because whenever these practices were written down, they were written in secret codes and allegories known only to insiders of the author's branch or lineage.

Old Taoist temples and communities were scattered over many regions. They were disparate groups that developed diverse beliefs and customs. That is why Taoism today has many branches with widely different philosophies and practices. Most of these branches offer wisdom from the old monks mixed with regional superstitions of more primitive religions from long ago. That's why some branches and their practices closely resemble sorcery or pantheism, while others focus on meditation and natural lifestyle, and still others focus on ritual and worship. Each sect picked up local or regional religious customs and blended them with their own practice. As the centuries passed, Taoism rubbed up against other prevailing religious beliefs, such as those of Confucianism, Buddhism, and others, and these encounters added even more layers of custom and ritual to certain segments of today's Taoist practice.

This is one reason why the old true wisdom from the original monks is only partially preserved within the layers of rituals found in the practices of modern Taoism. The fundamental meaning, purpose, and transformative power behind most of these rituals have unfortunately been lost through general misunderstanding and the mixing with other religions and philosophical views. The true teachings of the ancient monks—and even Taoism itself—almost vanished completely at certain junctures in history due to wave upon wave of political changes, wars, and power struggles in China. Regime changes sometimes resulted in many temples being burned to the ground and their masters and monks killed or forced into hiding.

In many cases, the real understanding of chi—how to work with it to reach that spark of yuan chi inside us and build a bridge back to the One Universal Energy of Tao—has been reduced to theories, speculations, and arcane practices with no explanations. That is why most people who seek the real practice to restore life energy find only its footprint in Taoism's many rituals and arts.

That's why I tell my students, "Ritual usually represents a failure of the truth." What does this mean? When we seek, learn, and then ultimately go through the repetitive motions and behaviors of rituals without having a deep understanding and experience of the power and meaning and purpose behind them, the truth remains lost to us. I warn students not to let their own practice become only ritual but to hold on to the true goal and purpose in their chi gung, t'ai chi, and Tao gung.

Unfortunately, much of today's teaching on these practices, while well meaning, is actually just passing along a ritual—a slow-motion exercise. You can learn the forms and postures and even experience some great results, but without the keys to the real goal of chi gung, t'ai chi, and Tao gung, and without the guidance of a master, you'll never come close to experiencing the true potential of these moving meditation practices.

In this book, we are interested in breaking away the outer shell of the rituals of those old Taoist meditation practices and teachings and pulling out the how-to marrow. We want to employ those teachings with full understanding so we can transform ourselves and restore our chi. We want to grab that thin thread of truth underneath the ancient teachings and practices, the thread that winds backward and links us to those monks who really knew how to restore their life energy and connect to the dimension of energy that powers the entire universe.

The good news is that this truth and practice are both very simple. What I'm about to share with you is easy to understand, and the practices are easy to learn. On the other hand, rising above your current condition and modern lifestyle to actually practice these simple truths can be extremely difficult. Persevering until you experience real and lasting change can be harder still. But the rewards you will receive by making this effort to restore your chi are so great that it is well worth your while.

The greatest adventure you will ever embark on is the journey back to the awareness of your original life energy. *Restoring Your Life Energy* is a map that will help take you there. I was lucky, as a young teenager, to be thrown together with an old monk at our local temple. He was a relic, a dinosaur of that long-lost, forgotten age of true Taoist wisdom. He was able to point me in the right direction, back to the center of my own life energy, despite my doubting, arrogant adolescent mind. I was fortunate enough to grab the tail of this dinosaur, this old tradition, and drag it forward so I can give it to whoever is interested.

In this book, we'll often stop to consider words from the most famous of the Taoist monks, Lao Tzu. Five hundred years before the birth of Christ, he gave us a short collection of Taoist wisdom called the *Tao Te Ching*. This book has been printed, translated, and interpreted all over the world for centuries, surpassed in popularity by only a few other books, such as the Bible. It's made up of eighty-one chapters that are often only a paragraph or two in length. Even though it is such a short work, Lao Tzu gets to the heart of how-to: how to restore our life energy and how to connect back to the Tao. But his words are not always easy to understand.

For example, scholars have traditionally misinterpreted even the meaning of the title. They translated *Tao Te Ching* as *The Book of Virtue*. In Chinese, when you combine the words *Tao* and *Te,* they become an adjective describing a high level of good conduct. You might pay a compliment to someone by saying, "He has a lot of tao-te," meaning he is a good, moral, and honorable person. Given this translation, scholars over the centuries have been trying to understand the *Tao Te Ching* as a guidebook for virtuous conduct. But that's not really what it is about at all.

Chinese words can have multiple meanings. That is part of the beauty, poetry, and mystery of the language. In fact, *Tao Te Ching* really means something much deeper. *Ching* means "book"; that's simple enough. *Tao* means the One Universal Energy and the Way that One Universal Energy works. Again, we might call this God in our culture today.

Te is that very special word we just talked about. Its original meaning refers to the piece of Tao, or God, inside each of us, that spark of original energy, the germ of life, that underlies and supports our chi. Because of this, our Te is the deepest, truest, most integral part of us. Do you see how this could be misinterpreted as virtue? Can you see the subtle difference?

What the words *Tao, Te,* and *Ching* really mean when they are put together in the title is, "Here's the book about the Tao and Te, the true energy outside and the true energy inside, the God out there and the piece of God inside." This book is an important resource for any journey to restore life energy. If you get the chance, you might want to read it. There are many translations out there. Pick up a few, look them over, and buy one you especially like. Even though the *Tao Te Ching* can seem strange and hard to understand at first, with a few re-readings and what you'll learn in this book, Lao Tzu's words will become clearer to you.

As you actually restore your chi, these mysterious words will make even more sense. Why? Because we are going to use this old wisdom and these old practices to chisel down into that pure and powerful part of you that understands everything effortlessly. We are going to use chi gung to dig down as close as possible to that Te inside you so you can restore your life energy.

I

CHI

Integral to Health and Peace of Mind

TO SEE THE MIRACLE of life energy, all we have to do is consider a seed. It's so small, so shriveled and dry. It's hard to believe that such a small thing can explode into something as large and full of life as a tree.

A seed and a tree look so different from each other. Unless somebody taught you the basics of botany or biology, you wouldn't even know that the two have any possible relationship to one another, much less that they are in some sense the same thing.

The seed and the tree are simultaneously completely different and completely connected. The miracle bridging the two is a mysterious and invisible force—the *life energy* deep inside the seed. It's that miracle of intelligent force, that constructive blueprint, that power that explodes into the first green shoot after a spring rain, that quiet wisdom that governs the entire process of a seed growing into a tree that later produces more seeds. We cannot see it, we cannot hear it, we cannot taste or smell it. We can only observe its monumental effects by the evidence of the towering tree standing in front of us.

The life energy of the seed is the same life that creates the leaves, the sap, the fruit, the bark, and the wood of the tree. It is the same life energy that tells the tree when to grow new buds and when to drop its leaves and go dormant for the winter. It gives the tree its "consciousness" in its own world of sun, water, wind, and soil. Everything in, on, and about that tree depends on and is linked together by that same invisible life energy. And absolutely all of that tree's power and potential was inherent in that original, dry, dead-looking seed.

Did you know you have a lot in common with the seed and the tree? You, too, sprang from a tiny seed—the seed we call the first single cell. From that microscopic beginning, over a long and miraculous journey, that single cell made the astounding transformation into an embryo, a fetus, and then a newborn. Since your birth, the original energy from your first single cell continues to explode into the full-grown human being you are today, with all your talents, strengths, and capabilities. That same energy is what still enlivens and sustains. Just like that journey from a seed to a tree, the journey from that single cell into who you are now is made possible by the original intelligence, power, and blueprint held within your life energy.

Your life energy was smart and industrious enough to pull in all the necessary building blocks to create your body. It established the flow of blood through your veins; it created your brain; it enlivens your organs and tells them what to do; it fuels your mind and thought processes; and it produces your consciousness, which enables your spirit to function. Without that energy, your body would fall limp, your brain would cease to function, and your spirit could no longer maintain its connection to your body. This same life energy—carried forward from that first single cell—creates, sustains, and holds every part of you together: from top to bottom, inside and out.

Clearly, if such a small amount of life energy can do so much, it is a precious substance. If such energy is what builds, maintains, and fuels the mind, body, and spirit, it is clear that we must protect and cherish it.

But the sad fact is that from the moment we emerge from the womb, our life energy—chi—starts to weaken, becoming vulnerable to contamination and distortion. That's why we age, suffer, experience illness, and eventually die. Our chi loses its integrity.

As newborns we are like brand-new cars with zero miles. As infants and young children, our bodies run smoothly, and our chi is able to repair itself and any injuries seamlessly and quickly. But as we age, we rack up more and more miles. Pretty soon breakdowns are inevitable. We lose our original integrity of function, just like old cars. If only we could turn back the odometer and restore the pristine purity of that newborn chi.

We can, but it takes work. In today's society, few people are even aware that they have something called chi, or life energy. They take it for granted and don't consider that this special part of themselves is worth learning about, strengthening, and protecting.

Modern life has us chasing many outward goals: happiness, riches, fame, success, security, career satisfaction, friends, family, entertainment, and so on. We rarely take the time to stop, look inward, and take stock of the condition of our chi. Like old cars, we keep on driving and take it for granted until something breaks down. Only then do we wish we'd paid more attention to maintenance.

Understandably, we want all the joys that life can give us, so we keep trying for more. We work, strive, chase, and study to achieve goals that will give us more money, more enjoyment, more prestige, more friends—more, more, more. Who has time to stop and look within? To stop and meditate or repair or even remember that we have something as vague and subtle as life energy?

It's as if everyone wants to live like a millionaire. Let's consider what that means. A person with lots of success, many friends, and a wealth of riches increases his sense of worth in our world. We'll represent him with the number 1,000,000. As he accumulates more wealth, more family, more friends, more power, and more prestige, it's as if he keeps adding more and more zeroes to the increasing sum of his life worth. He may even become 1,000,000,000. A person with more modest life achievements might only be seen as 1,000. Who wants to be just 1,000 or 100? Give us more zeroes!

The problem is that we keep wanting to add more good things, chasing more and more zeroes, to increase our sense of worth, but we never stop to consider the condition of our number one. Our life energy is like the number one to all of those zeroes. What happens to the number 1,000 or 1,000,000 or 1,000,000,000 if you take away the one at the beginning? They each become nothing. While we may feel like millionaires, if we don't keep and protect that number one, we risk being left with only a string of zeroes.

Instead of chasing more zeroes to add to your life sum, it is wiser to look after and protect your one. After all, Lao Tzu asks in the *Tao Te Ching,* "What is more important, your wealth or your life?"

He also urges those who seek the Tao to "embrace the One." He's not referring to embracing merely our own life energy. He's actually saying to embrace the One Power of Tao. But to embrace the Tao, you have to start by being able to embrace your own life energy, to put it first in your life. How can you hope to embrace the Tao if you cannot find, feel, protect, and embrace your own chi, the piece of Tao inside you?

If you go back and read the U.S. Declaration of Independence, you'll find the hallmark statement that all people "are endowed by their creator with certain inalienable rights, that among these are life, liberty, and the pursuit of happiness." The founding fathers showed a lot of wisdom. Life must come first, for without it, how can we enjoy liberty? Without life, the pursuit of happiness is meaningless. To protect liberty, happiness, and anything else we value, we must first protect *life.* And that means protecting and preserving the integrity of our life energy.

Today, we've lost sight of our real priorities. You can go to many time management seminars or even buy special life-planning notebooks that help you set your priorities and get the most out of your day. But if you were to sneak a peak at most people's daily list of priorities and life goals, it's probable that almost none would include protecting and strengthening their chi.

Whoever you are, whatever you are doing right now, let's erase everything else for just a little while and put life energy at the top of your priority list. Let's invest a little time to learn more about this invisible but powerful force inside. Let's discover a way to nourish and preserve it. After all, it's the most precious treasure we possess. If you agree, it's time we unwrap that treasure and take a look.

2

HOW CHI GETS DAMAGED, WEAKENED, OR BLOCKED

THE HUMAN BODY is a miraculous creation. From one tiny cell, it grows into an amazing conscious being with a phenomenal body that was meant to be a rechargeable, self-repairing, self-defending living energy system. One could argue that, by original design, human beings were meant to live forever. What went wrong? Why do we age, get sick, and die? Why does our living energy system wear out and run down? The simple answer is because our chi loses its strength and integrity.

To restore our life energy, we must first understand how it functions inside us and how it gets damaged. When we can understand, reduce, or even remove the damaging influences to our chi, we've taken a big step toward healing and restoring it.

HOW DOES CHI WORK?

Chi is the invisible life energy that flows through invisible channel-like meridians throughout your body. You won't necessarily find these energy meridians if you dissect a human body, but you can map them and even measure the chi flowing through them with sensitive electronic instruments. These meridians and the flow of chi are what acupuncturists,

Chinese herbalists, and energy healers endeavor to treat. They try to repair weakness, blockages, excess, and imbalances in your chi.

On a simple level, we can compare our life energy to electricity flowing through a wire or grid. If electricity flows through a faulty or kinked wire, or if the circuits in the grid get overloaded or crossed, the flow of energy can become weakened, excessive, or blocked. The same thing happens when the flow of chi is blocked or weakened; it hurts our health and well-being. So we can work to get the kinks out of the wire, repairing our grid to make sure the energy is flowing through the correct circuits in the right direction at just the right voltage. This is how Chinese medicine tries to work. It restores the correct flow through the right meridians or channels in the right amount at the right time.

Using electricity is a simple analogy to help us understand chi, but it's not the whole story. When we compare chi to electricity, the analogy falls short. Life energy isn't just a *quantity* of power, like kilowatts of electricity, that we can meter and steer through a circuit; life energy also has *quality* and content. Chi can carry an energy signal. This means that, in addition to power, it also contains programming, content, and message. So instead of comparing life energy to electricity, we should say it's more like the energy of television or radio waves.

When a television broadcast comes flowing across the airwaves or through a cable to your television screen, it not only has energy, it has content. And that content matters to you. If the energy signal flowing into your television contains an episode of *I Love Lucy,* both the result on your screen and your viewing experience are much different than if the energy contains a replay of a horror movie like *Friday the 13th.* To consider those television waves as simply energy or power flowing through the air or a wire is missing an important truth. That energy can carry a wide variety of different programming that delivers different results in the end.

Much of our chi damage occurs because our life energy picks up the wrong "program" and then carries that program throughout our system. Originally, our chi carried the pure and original program with which we came into this world—the signal of the pure, creative life force we enjoyed when we were a single cell. That's the signal that most closely matches the signal from the original energy of the Universe. That's the signal we want. That's also why infants and children are usually quite healthy, carefree, spontaneous, and centered. They still have that original program pulsing loud and strong through their life energy.

As we grow up, year by year, our chi picks up a lot of outside information that changes that pure inner signal over time. Instead of the original programming (a program of health, restoration, nourishment, and harmony), our adult energy becomes infected with wrong programming that distorts our life energy signal.

The body thrives when it receives that pure original signal; it struggles without it. That's why we adults endure more stress, illness, anxiety, and disharmony than children: the wrong signals that now infect our chi are carried and broadcast to each cell in our body and mind, causing distortion, decline, and suffering.

This is why we need to work on restoring the right signal to our chi. Much of our meditation and the chi gung practices we will discuss is aimed at reprogramming our life energy to that pure original signal that allows us to thrive. We need to turn up the signal of that original program of pure life energy so our chi can once again carry it to every cell of our body and mind.

CHI: THE MIND-BODY BRIDGE

Chi not only enlivens the body, it also fuels the consciousness. For that reason, it serves as a bridge between the mind and body. It's the medium, the messenger, the highway of energy information that coordinates the mind and body. It is the backbone of all that we now refer to as mind-body health and wellness.

That information bridge is why holding sad or angry thoughts in your mind can actually create physical sensations in your gut or even cause damage to your body over time. Conversely, when your physical body is ill or injured, that same bridge can influence your mind and mood to feel sad, depressed, and unmotivated. Your chi has the ability to carry messages instantaneously from your mind to your body and from your body to your mind.

Chi is not only the bridge between the mind and body; it is the bridge between the mind and the outside world. It's chi that makes the mind and its activity, including the use of the five senses, possible. It's the mind and those five senses that go outside to touch, smell, communicate, see, and hear everything going on outside us. After all, isn't our consciousness and the ability to sense and experience things what we really value and define as *life*?

It's not because we have a brain and a nose and two eyes that we are able to experience our world; it's because we have chi. That conscious life energy is what allows our mind and senses to experience and interact with the outside world. A cadaver has a brain and a nose and two eyes. But without that chi, it cannot experience anything.

WHAT DAMAGES CHI?

Poor-quality chi, or chi that carries a bad signal, can damage our system, causing illness or even death. There are four main factors that contribute to bad programming in our life energy. They lead to damaged and weakened chi, no matter how we might try to conserve, repair, or recharge it. These four factors are mind activity, artificial concepts, negative impact, and previous use.

MIND ACTIVITY AND ARTIFICIAL CONCEPTS

When we are a single cell, a fetus, or a newborn, we don't use our mind to interpret our world. We don't think about our surroundings. We simply experience everything by true, whole, spontaneous feeling. However, as we grow from infancy to adulthood, we rely more and more on our mind to collect and interpret our experiences of the world.

When our mind makes interpretations about our experiences, we get into trouble. These interpretations are really just artificial notions. We can make them up in our head, or we can pick them up from others. Nonetheless, such interpretations are always artificial. Then we choose to add these artificial interpretations to a whole collection of other artificial interpretations we carry around in our mind.

We add more and more to the collection with each new experience and every passing day. The accumulation of these notions and interpretations, and how we manipulate them in our mind, is called thinking. Thinking is actually very artificial when compared to the true, direct, and spontaneous experience of life through the direct feeling of our life energy that we enjoyed as infants.

That's why thinking puts us at risk for contaminating our chi with the wrong programming. Thinking is removed and separate, not real. It's based on manufactured ideas about the world around us. It may or may not have anything to do with the actual truth and the real, present-moment experience of the world. Thinking is ultimately and always only partial truth.

As adults, we are full of judgments, rights and wrongs, and predigested interpretations. We've built a complicated, unreal world inside our thinking mind. We "experience" the world only after our senses pass through our mind's labyrinth of preconceptions and interpretations. This bears no resemblance to the direct experience of a baby.

What's worse, we elevate the importance of our thinking and our so-called knowledge. We consider it more reliable than the direct experience of our chi. We look down on an infant who simply grabs a toy and puts it in her mouth, focusing all of her attention on that single moment of sensation. We consider ourselves smart in comparison.

But all of the artificial thoughts and judgments we carry in our thinking overwhelm, outshout, and eventually separate us from our original life energy signal. These wrong programs begin to dominate the content of our chi so that we can no longer hear or feel that beneficial, balancing, and pure original program.

As adults, we pride ourselves on our education. The more education we receive, the more intelligent we consider ourselves to be. We worship and respect those experts who have lists of higher degrees after their names. But education merely yields a larger and larger collection of predigested, artificial interpretations. We have more junk clogging up our thinking and separating us from the pure unbiased mind of our original life energy.

In the *Tao Te Ching*, Lao Tzu warned about the dubious value of so-called knowledge and education:[1]

> Washing and cleansing your mind to obtain the true original vision, can you be without contamination?
>
> Give up learning and become worry-free.
>
> Shut your knowledge; close the door of your cleverness.
>
> Learn how not to need to learn, to avoid repeating others' mistakes.

> Those who know the truth possess no knowledge. Those who possess knowledge do not know the truth.

He knew that when we focus on our thinking, it keeps us in a world of artificial ideas. Such artificial knowledge keeps us away from truth, because it keeps us from feeling, connecting with, and using the direct experience of our original life energy.

Lao Tzu wants us to return to a better way. Instead of stuffing our mind with artificial interpretations, he wants us to use our pure mind, our absolute mind in its original state—like the mind of a baby. In our mind's original state, there are no value judgments, no artificial meanings, no rehearsed interpretations or formulas.

Relying on life energy instead of your knowledge doesn't make you dumb and stupid. Far from it! That original life energy holds the infinite power and intelligence of the universe. Instead, your mind in its original state can instantly contact that core of Te inside you and just "know." When you get closer to that real energy, you'll get the correct signal of what the truth is in every situation and know instinctively and automatically what to do. You won't need any education to figure things out when you have access to your original energy.

That's why Lao Tzu described the man who can connect to Te as able to stay inside all day and, without even looking out his window, know everything in the entire world. He can do this just by connecting to that original intelligent energy of the Universe. That piece of Tao, your Te, is connected to the entire net of original energy that extends across the universe. When you touch that Te, you touch the entire net.

Here's the irony: you can only get closer to touching that net—that original, infinite intelligence—by using the pure mind of a baby. No amount of education or learning will help you reach it. Your everyday, artificial, thinking mind cannot connect to the original energy of the Tao. Only pure absolute mind has that ability. Staying mired in your thinking and knowledge keeps you closed off from that original signal.

At every juncture in life, we are trained to turn to thought, the artificial collection of junk in our brain, for the answer. We are never trained to turn to the feeling of our life energy, the source of truth, for the answer. So we keep going in the wrong direction, adding to our knowledge, walling ourselves off from the Te inside.

So by favoring our thinking as much as we do, not only do we pick up wrong programming, we gradually strangle off that original and natural connection to the Te that is our birthright. We ignore it for so long that our ability to hear what our original energy wants and needs atrophies. The Te inside says, "Oh, you don't need me anymore? Okay, go ahead and use your thinking. I'll hide here and go to sleep." It's as if our original energy signal goes into hibernation.

It requires hard work to wake up that ability again. It starts by learning how to bypass your reliance on artificial thinking. Then you must begin using the pure vehicle of sincere feeling to restore the ability to feel your chi. It's like using a muscle that hasn't been used for a long time. It takes practice, exercise, and time to regain what you've lost.

So the first step in slowing the damage to your chi is to reverse what you normally do. Instead of allowing thinking to block your life energy, you work to block your thinking in favor of feeling your life energy signal. With practice, persistence, and the internal healing work of chi gung, you can reawaken that correct energy signal and put it in charge once again.

NEGATIVE IMPACT

When the ancient monks and monastic orders encouraged people to keep their minds calm and to reduce their desires and interactions with the outside world, they were teaching them a way to protect their life energy. They were trying to help those seekers protect their internal programming. When we use our mind's thinking ability or send our mind and senses out into the world, we risk picking up bad programming that infects our chi.

How? A kid goes out in the backyard and runs around having fun, seeing and doing all sorts of things. But when you let a kid go outside, he comes back rumpled and dirty. His fingers, nose, and pants are all muddy.

Your mind is the same way. When it takes chi to fuel its senses and thinking and then goes out to interact with our artificial, crazy world, it can pick up a lot of bad interpretations and dirty signals. This crud can stay in your mind and cling to your life energy, sending an artificial or even damaging program to your entire system.

When your mind comes back from arguing with a friend, watching a horror movie, or reading all the bad news in the paper, it can come back contaminated with negative ideas, pictures, and interpretations. This contamination can infect and overpower your thinking for a long time. And because your thinking is fueled by and in ever-present contact with your chi, this means your chi can become muddy and infected too. That's how chi contamination can change your program, your life energy signal.

Remember that chi flows ceaselessly throughout your being, affecting every cell in your body as well as every mood and thought. Don't you want that chi to be as clean, calm, and pure as possible? Another tool to help restore your energy is reducing the risk of negative input.

But how can you keep your chi clean and uncontaminated by junk from outside? You can choose to reduce your contact with overtly negative people, situations, entertainment, and news. That does help, which is why Buddha used to ask his disciples, "Can you see no evil? Hear no evil? Speak no evil?" He understood how negative impact could undermine his disciples' progress by contaminating their minds and chi.

The type of lifestyle that sharply reduces exposure to negative input may have been far easier in those old Buddhist or Taoist temples. The monks deliberately kept themselves secluded so they could work on purifying their energy from the type of negative contamination found everywhere in public life. However, most of us live in the real world and cannot afford to re-create a protected, templelike environment. We can't help but be exposed to the negative stress of everyday life. Aside from living in a temple, what else can we do to prevent crud from sticking to our life energy?

Consider this: nothing sticks well to a surface that is clean and totally smooth. For something to stick, the surface needs to have grooves, imperfections, or receptors that the sticky material can cling to. Likewise, negative energy signals can only attach to you and stick to your life energy if you have receptors for those negative messages inside you.

Strong, intact chi has no receptors to which dirty energy can attach. That negative signal will just bounce or slide right off. It's because your chi is damaged that it becomes a receptor for and holds on to negative input. It's no longer smooth and strong. It has cavities, imperfections, and receptors that outside junk can latch onto. Of course, when you have junk clinging to your chi, it will in turn attract more junk—just like sticky or grooved surfaces in your kitchen attract more bacteria, dust, and debris. The more receptors you have, the more junk can cling to you, which in turn causes even more damage, which then creates more receptors, and so on. This sets up a negative feedback loop that leads to your demise.

We've already used a baby as a model of someone with strong, intact chi. What happens when you look directly into a baby's eyes, smile, lightly tickle his stomach, and say in a soft and playful voice, "You little jerk! You are so lousy. I hate you. Look how little and ugly you are." The baby doesn't care. Unless you are too loud, have a scary face, or hurt him physically, he will just gurgle and coo, laugh at you, and go back to sucking his toes. His pure mind has no receptor for your insults. That negative stuff cannot stick to him. But if you say and do exactly the same thing to an adult who has weak chi and relies on his mind to experience the world, you may wreak all sorts of damage and get a totally different reaction with those same words and behavior. You might even get punched in the nose.

You have to repair your life energy so you can be more like that baby. You want the onslaught of negative attacks from life in the modern world to have less effect on you. The good news is that you can smooth and clean your life energy through chi gung. With proper practice, you can eliminate those receptors for bad energy. Your practice serves as a grindstone, teaching you to focus, relax, and stay calm. Meanwhile, through the moving meditation of chi gung, you help your energy flow to keep it clean and pure and strong. Soon you can enjoy watching more and more of that bad stuff bounce right off you. Over time, through the benefits of your practice, you may not even notice or be bothered by situations that used to vex you in the past.

RECYCLED ENERGY

When you started life here on earth, you were a tiny single cell. Although you had tremendous power, you were still just that one cell. To grow and develop into the billions of cells you are today, that first cell had to acquire building material. You pulled in the physical building blocks you needed through the umbilical cord that connected you to your mother—proteins, enzymes, minerals, and water, all for the construction of your developing body.

All of that material had been used before. The protein used to construct your blood vessels may have come from a chicken sandwich your mother ate for dinner. Not long before, it was running around a barnyard as part of the chicken. The drop of water used to keep your cells hydrated may have originally been part of a river or pond, or it may have been drunk long ago by Abraham Lincoln. After old Abe used it, it returned to the water cycle to evaporate and condense a hundred times or more and rain back down into your city's water supply.

No matter where all this recycled material came from, your embryo gladly took it in, because you needed it in order to grow. You took whatever you could get, whatever was available to you, to keep building new cells. If your mother ate good-quality food and drank pure, clean water, you had a lucky break. If she took in junk, that's what you were forced to use.

In addition to pulling in the physical building blocks you needed, you also pulled in additional life energy to fuel and enliven these new cells. You had access to energy from your mother and her food, from the energy in the immediate environment, and even from the energy radiating down through whatever part of the universe the earth was traveling through at the time. This outside life energy you drew in and made part of yourself was also recycled. It was used before.

You see, energy in our universe is never destroyed. It simply changes form. The same is true for life energy. When we are finished with our life energy at the time of our death, it drops away like clothes we are finished wearing. Another person who needs clothes may come along and pick it up. The Tao wastes nothing. Everything is recycled.

Likewise, when an embryo needs to take in more life energy, it will pick up whatever has been left behind in the immediate vicinity. If there is clean, high-quality energy available, that's great! If not, then too bad, that embryo must still take whatever it can get.

No matter what its quality, all energy has been used somewhere and sometime before, in some form or other. Therefore, that energy the embryo picks up has a history. Because of its history, the energy comes with residue of past programming. It has a residual signal, an imprint, a memory.

When you drive a new car off the dealer's lot, it feels and smells new and has never been owned by anyone else. You may be its first driver, turning that odometer from zero to one. Nevertheless, chances are that many parts of that car came from recycled material. The engine block could be forged from steel that was once part of a faraway bridge. The axles may contain metal that was once part of an old bathtub. The window glass may be mixed from other glass that once served as milk or medicine bottles.

So although your new car is truly new and one of a kind and it has never before existed as one piece, some parts of it have been used before in other ways by other things. These parts have a history.

This is similar to your life energy. Bits and pieces of your chi come from the recycling bin. The difference between recycled life energy and recycled metal is that the former is alive! It thus becomes part of the overall chi flow inside you and infuses your entire body and mind with whatever leftover imprints it carries. That's why the history of the recycled life energy you are currently borrowing can keenly affect you today.

We can catch a glimpse of the effects of recycled energy as we grow up and discover individual preferences and aversions. A woman may find that for some reason she cannot resist shoplifting. She feels compelled to steal what she wants, even though she is smart enough to know this is unwise and she could get caught. What she may not realize is that her shoplifting urge is an echo of energy that was used before by a thief and is now part of her chi. A part of her energy carries that memory imprint of stealing, and that programming is now an interwoven part of her life energy signal.

Perhaps as she grows up, that same woman discovers she has a keen sense of tune and pitch. She loves music and cannot get enough of it. She easily plays any instrument she picks up. This talent may be from a bit of recycled energy in her chi that was once used by a musician long ago. It carries that imprint of musical appreciation and ability.

Other traditions may refer to these old imprints as karma or past lives. But the real way to understand this situation is to know that we now carry bits of energy that are recycled and have a history. That history can benefit us, or it can carry negative programming that can ultimately hurt us and distort our life energy. These old messages can be so strong and loud that they drown out our pure, original life energy signal, steering us into damaging actions that lead to illness, suffering, and ruin. That recycled energy can also end up serving as a receptor that attracts more bad stuff from outside.

So another process in restoring our life energy is working to scrub, burn off, and purify the old remnant echoes in that recycled energy so we can regain our true signal. We need to make our pure signal strong and loud.

Between all of our artificial thinking, the damaging noise of negative impact from outside, and the echoes of our recycled chi, it's no wonder we have a hard time hearing our original life energy signal. Right now the condition of the chi inside your body is a lot like a room with several dozen radios blaring different stations all at once. One of those radios is playing a beautiful symphony that your cells would love to hear, but they can't because of the interference and noise from all the other programs. If you want to hear that symphony, you need to go inside, walk around the room, and turn off—or at least turn down—the volume of all those other radios so you can find the one playing the beautiful symphony. Then you can grab that radio and turn up the volume so that symphony can fill the entire room

This is why purifying and cleaning our chi is an important part of restoring it. Chi gung, t'ai chi, and Tao gung help us with this task!

3

RESTORING THE LIFE ENERGY SIGNAL

WE'VE EXPLORED several ways in which life energy can be damaged by wrong programming and the sources of those wrong signals. Now we want to learn how to restore our pure, original, and correct signal.

How do you find the right signal? A good question to ask: "When was my life energy at its most pure, powerful, and original state?"

Sometimes when I teach, I ask my students to show me a photo of themselves: "Give me the picture that shows the true you at your best." Most will pull out photos that show them as smart, successful young adults, good-looking and full of accomplishments.

But I wonder why nobody chooses their baby picture—"That's me. Look how cute I am, Master!" After all, in many ways, a baby picture is a better representation of the real you before you acquired all the fake interpretations and problems that dominate your life today. Your life energy was strong, fresh, and new. Your mind was untroubled. Your body was supple and self-regulating. However, most people disregard a baby photo: "Nah. Why would that picture represent me? I was so stupid, small, and weak."

I would be very impressed indeed if someone could bring me a picture of him- or herself as a single cell in the womb. It's almost too disturbing to consider that you and I and every person on this planet spent at least twenty minutes or so as a single cell. We don't want to think of ourselves like that, because we consider a single cell to be insignificant, vulnerable, and weak. Yet if you could carry a picture of that cell in your wallet, it would be no less *you* than the attractive, professional portrait you staple to your résumé.

The real truth is that our life energy signal was at its purest, strongest, and most original state when we were that one original cell. If we could tap into the pure potential and power we had as that cell, our life energy would instantly have the original pattern for perfect health and function for each part of our body.

Think of it, inside that single cell was the original blueprint for a perfectly functioning heart, liver, brain, and digestive system. Inside it was the intelligent ability to pull in every protein, enzyme, and physical building block needed to create every tissue of our body correctly.

There was even enough original power in that cell to split itself into two without any assistance. Can you do that? Can you stand there with all your adult strength and education and pull yourself apart into two new perfectly whole and functioning selves? Now if you had lots of muscle, nerves of steel, and a large pole to grab, you might be able to pull against yourself hard enough to dislocate your own shoulder. But your original cell split in two with no leverage, nothing to brace itself against, nothing to hold on to. It split while floating in liquid. The magnitude of such power and innate intelligence is amazing! And all within a cell no bigger than the head of a pin.

That first split was so powerful, it was like a "big bang" that left a permanent record in your body. The line down the middle of your torso, both front and back, is a scar or mark from that original split. Your torso looks like it's round, but inside you are more like two joined cylinders, reminiscent of those first two cells. That's why you have two of everything—two arms, two legs, two eyes, two ears, and so on.

That single cell not only had the power and programming to duplicate itself over and over again into exactly what was needed for every inch of your body, most of what it created was self-repairing. Through the long and miraculous nine months between your physical conception and birth, each newly created cell knew exactly what to do to harmonize and communicate with all the other differentiated cells at each phase of development from embryo to fetus to infant.

What if you had that kind of strength and power available to you in everyday life? Do you think you'd have more energy to handle your day? Could you address the problems in your life more effectively? Would your health and sense of well-being improve?

This is why medical science is now looking to stem cells for healing miracles. It realizes the potential, power, and intelligent life energy inherent in those original cells. It knows that cells closer to the time of prenatal development have much more restorative potential. What you need to realize is that the first single cell that was once you was the ultimate and original stem cell.

Understanding the power of that single cell is important. Why? Because losing that power is one of the reasons why we age, get ill, and die. You see, your cells must be able to divide and reproduce for your body to heal and repair itself. What is aging? Ultimately, it is the loss of cells' ability to divide and replicate properly. If your cells replicate too slowly, your body wears down. If they replicate irregularly, you lose function in your organs and tissues. If replication spins wildly out of control, you get cancer. If your cells stop replicating, you die.

Now do you see why you ought to be very interested in the power and programming of that single cell? Such power is the regulator and sustainer of health, youthfulness, and life. It pulses with that original pure signal and programming we've been talking about. It is that power that is a microcosm, a copy, a mirror of the power of the Tao itself.

The good news is that you still have that original single cell signal, or at least the memory of it, deep inside you. After all, the cell division process still occurs inside you millions of times each day. Even better news is that there is an ancient path preserving the steps of how to find that power, tap into it, and reincorporate it into your life. It's that power we are mimicking and seeking to wake up through chi gung.

THE POWERFUL THIRD FORCE

In the year 300 A.D., many centuries before it acquired the name *t'ai chi* from Master Chang San Feng in the thirteenth century, or chi gung from common usage, the earliest Taoist temples were using moving meditation for life energy and spiritual development. In these early stages, some practitioners had a very interesting name for it: *prenatal meditation*. Through such meditation, they worked to reach a state similar to what we experienced before we were born. This moving meditation was designed to wake up that long-forgotten memory hidden within and to coax that original life energy signal to come out and become dominant once again.

Perhaps you've seen the universal symbol for t'ai chi:

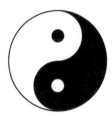

Does it remind you of that cellular activity we've been talking about? That first cell dividing into two? The power of the first cell division is the miraculous power of original life energy and a mirror of the power of the Tao itself.

But the wisdom behind the t'ai chi symbol doesn't end there. We can see the black and the white inside it, but there is also a third power hidden in that symbol. Can you see it? It is the curved line separating and connecting the black and white halves, holding them together and giving the symbol a sense of motion. You cannot see it, but without it, the symbol would fall apart.

Lao Tzu says in the *Tao Te Ching,*

> The Tao created the one. The one flows into two. The two generate the three. And the third kind of power at work begot the ten thousand things.[1]

This is just like what happens in your first cell. The force of life is created in that single cell that through the power of flow splits in two. At this instant, a third power is created between and around the two new cells. It grows as the cells continue to multiply. The third force is your chi.

As the curved line in the diagram, the chi holds each part together and coordinates their harmonious, ongoing movement. It's also the chi that holds your cells together and keeps them communicating with each other. It's that third force that sends certain cells off to the right to make your liver and others to the left to form your spleen. It directs nutrients to go where they're needed. It detects invaders and sends the immune system to attack. It governs which cells have to be sacrificed for the good of the whole. Through its harmonizing, communication, and management power, it creates Lao Tzu's ten thousand things.

It's the power of the third force that keeps billions of new cells together to comprise one functioning living being. Without that force, the internal organs could not work in concert. There would be billions of isolated and independent cells with no connection to each other, no harmony, no communication. It would be every cell for itself.

This aggregating third force has the ability to communicate to all the cells in your body and also penetrate and contact the original power *within* your cells. That's why, although it is invisible and subtle, the state of your chi is of paramount importance to you. Since it flows everywhere throughout your body and mind, if that third force is weak or carries a bad message, it can negatively affect each and every cell of your body at a deep level. That weak or faulty message can damage your health, your peace of mind, and your spiritual condition. This is why we want to connect to, purify, and strengthen your chi through chi gung.

OUR BACKWARD JOURNEY

What's the answer to restoring our chi to the power and pure signal of our original life energy? We start by learning where we *won't* find the answer. We won't find it outside ourselves. People have forever been looking outside themselves for the answers to life, health, peace, and meaning. They look in books, look to religions, look to masters and gurus, mediums and prophets. But the most powerful answer they seek is right inside them. Every person's answers are within the power of that original life energy signal inside.

In our lives, we may accumulate much knowledge, many accomplishments, and even some degree of spiritual understanding. We like to think we are always evolving and congratulate ourselves on that fact. We like the idea of moving onward, upward, and forward. We believe that our ultimate goals are always ahead of us or require attaining more from outside ourselves.

What we don't realize is that while we think we are going forward, we are never actually evolving but constantly devolving. Why? Because from the moment we are born, we begin to move further away from the pure power and potential inherent in that original germ of life inside our original cell. The further *forward* we go, the fainter that signal of life energy and harmony becomes, exerting less nourishing influence on us.

On our journey to restore chi, we are not moving forward to look outside ourselves in hopes of gaining anything new. We aren't seeking anything we don't already have. Instead, we are trying to go back to the amazing power, purity, and oneness of when we were a single cell. On the journey to restore our chi, the more we rely on our accumulated gains in life, the more we lose in respect to our life energy. Indeed, what we think we gain as we move forward in life can actually hurt us if it compounds the layer upon layer of insulation sealing us off from our original life energy signal.

Our journey is not forward—it's *backward*! If our life energy signal devolves as we age, we must go backward to restore it. We want to be able to put our body back to its original way of being, the way it was before we were born.

To go backward, we need to learn how to strip away what insulates us from connecting with our life energy. We need to withdraw our focus from all the artificial thoughts and concerns in life that replace or distract us from this goal. In our practice, we may only be able to accomplish this for a few seconds or a few minutes, but that's enough to start working our way backward.

You see, we are like computers. When we are new, we run fast and clean. But the more software we install, the slower our computer gets and the further away from that original streamlined operation. To restore our computer, we need to strip away old and useless programs; we need to reduce the amount of software and scrub the hard drive. We need to go backward to a restore point, a time when the hard drive was more pristine, before it got contaminated with all those viruses and bad programs.

This concept of going backward separates the true teaching of chi from many other spiritual teachings today. We are not working to transcend, transform, or evolve higher and further away from what we are now, going to a distant goal on a linear journey forward. We are not reaching up and out to move further outside ourselves for our answers. No, we must instead go backward and transform ourselves by reconnecting with the power and memory of that pure single cell within.

Why? Because backward and inward is where the spark of pure life, our Te, that piece of God inside us, lies. It's at the very center of our being. We must return to that center. That's the part of us that is our True Self. It's the part that entered this dimension from the dimension of Origin, God, or Tao. If we can go backward and return to that center, then all wisdom, true power, and real transformation is ours. Backward is the way to the evolution we really need.

That's what those old monks in the temples were really trying to do. They were trying to go backward to the point at which life began. They believed if they could go backward and touch the power of that single cell, they could then go even further backward through the gateway of life and death and return to the universal dimension where life first entered that cell. They had little or no interest in what lay outside them. Their journey was one of *returning.*

This is why the ancient temples created a lifestyle of reduction. They required members to strip away everything from the artificial, man-made world. When you entered the temple, they shaved your head and gave you a new name; you relinquished all your possessions; and you walked away from your family and your past. This was done to rid you of all distractions, to remove those things that drew you outward or mired you in artificial thinking, so you could focus inward and have a better chance of connecting with that powerful piece of God inside you. It also served as a symbolic act to remind you of the original truth. It said that the "real" person is not found in any of those outward facets of life, nor is it found in the artificial world. The real person is what's inside.

The old monks tried to establish a lifestyle that would help them reach their ultimate goal. They knew that the gateway of life and death—the gate through which original life energy enters this dimension and becomes that first single cell—is very, very small. You cannot go through that gateway carrying a lot of junk. You won't fit! Only what is refined, pure, and original can fit through that gate. So the monks worked diligently to strip away everything in their minds, their lives, and their energy that wasn't pure, absolute truth, or part of that signal of original Te.

Lao Tzu remarks in the *Tao Te Ching,*

> In the pursuit of studying world affairs, every day your knowledge accumulates. In the pursuit of Tao, every day you abandon. You abandon more—you reduce.[2]

This journey of restoring your chi will be unlike any other self-help or spiritual journey you've ever taken. On this journey, you are not seeking anything "new." You are not trying to gain anything outside yourself. Instead, you are working to reduce what you have learned; reduce outside distractions; and rediscover, regain, and employ something you've always had. You're going to travel backward to bring back all that old, lost, ignored, discarded feeling memory of chi buried deep within you.

4

MAKING THE CHI CONNECTION
FOR HEALTH

"BUT I TAKE CARE of my life energy," you're saying. "I'm very health conscious. I keep up on all the latest research and wellness advice to keep my body healthy and strong."

That's great. However, taking care of your health by conventional means isn't the same as taking care of your life energy. Your physical health and your life energy certainly affect each other, but they aren't quite the same thing.

Your body is more like a horse that you ride through your life. The real *you* is the rider. See the difference?

Am I saying your body is not important? Not at all! Many religions like to separate the soul and the body so they can elevate the soul while they downplay, dismiss, or even despise the body. This is very unwise. If your body is the horse you ride through life, you'd better take good care of that horse!

I've met lots of people who own stables and horses. It's funny, but many of these people take far better care of their horses than they do their own bodies. They give their horses only the best feed in calculated amounts, special vitamins, and just the right amount of exercise every day. They bathe and groom their horses and hire special doctors to look them over on a regular basis. They may even have a special swimming pool built just for their horses to exercise in.

But when you look at the owners, they may be in terrible condition: smoking, overweight and out of shape, wheezing, and maintaining a high-stress lifestyle. But there they are, pointing with pride across the pasture at their gleaming thoroughbreds. It's a mystery to me why they don't take any of the same measures they use to care for their horses to care for themselves.

In our case, with our body as the horse, we really need to take care of it, because guess what? If we take that horse for granted and never stop to give it what it needs, some day it will get sick, fall over, or die. Then what? We're in trouble. No more horse, no more life on this earth. Our life energy needs that horse.

Taking care of our health isn't as easy as it seems. Even those who try to be disciplined and health conscious still get sick and injured. Why? One reason is that our polluted and vulnerable minds have trouble discerning which health advice is good for us and which is not. That's the high price we pay when we rely on our mind and go outside for answers instead of inside to our life energy.

Our chi knows *exactly* what our body needs and how to repair it. The trouble is we never learn to connect to our life energy so we can ask and hear what it needs. Instead, we run to our data bank of artificial knowledge—we go to the library, consult the Internet, or find experts to tell us what to do. We bypass our life energy and put fitness trainers, special diets, pills, and medical procedures in charge of our body's delicate mechanisms of balance. So rather than cooperating with our life energy and giving it what it needs, we often work against it without even knowing it.

Did you ever notice how health advice changes over time? One month, the experts tell us, "Eat this." A few months later, they tell us, "Don't eat this; eat that instead." Miracle pills that are advertised on television one day are recalled from the shelves for causing harmful side effects a year later. But because we are so desperate to improve our health, we put our trust in this ever-changing and often contradictory world of health advisers. We put our very life in their hands—in addition to lots of money. When we lay down our life and wealth and obey an outside force unquestioningly, it's almost as if we are worshipping a god! But we have to be careful not to worship the wrong god when it comes to our health.

We need to learn and respect that the original life energy in our body knows exactly what is wrong and how to fix it. After all, it is a tiny copy of the Tao, the Universal Energy, or the real God. That's what we should listen to. We carry it inside us. It is working as our chief physician every second of every day, desperately trying to balance our body and restore our health. It is struggling to communicate with us, to tell us what we need to do so we can help ourselves. The trouble is that we can't hear it. That still, small voice is overwhelmed by all the other noise inside and outside.

MAKING THE CHI CONNECTION

We are all busy in our daily lives, running around, dazzled and impressed by the myriad outside information and activities the world offers. But all those distractions make it easy to forget that inside each and every one of us, right here and right now, is a miraculous and amazing living truth.

Many of my students come to learn t'ai chi from me so they can become martial artists. I tell them, "Listen, you already have martial arts ability inside you. You are a martial artist every second of every day. Why? Your immune system! It defends you expertly, defeating attacks every day."

Other students tell me they want to learn t'ai chi to become healers. I tell them, "You're already a healer. Your life energy is continually building new cells, tearing down old ones, removing poison, and delivering nutrition to every part of your body. It's all going on inside you."

That's why, before I teach my students anything else, I point them inside themselves to get in touch with that energy.

It's okay to look outside for answers about how to balance a checkbook, cook a casserole, or build a porch. However, relying only on outside advice to take care of our personal health is often a gamble. Sometimes outside advice will work because we have accidentally and luckily found what our chi needs to balance our body. But other times the advice will backfire because the treatment we or our doctors choose conflicts with and hinders the healing our chi is quietly but desperately trying to do inside. That's why sometimes a doctor's help works wonders and sometimes it doesn't.

The real answer to our problems is to restore our *chi awareness* and, through our chi, to increase our sensitivity to what our original energy is trying to tell us. We need to let our life energy be the boss.

Am I telling people to avoid doctors? No. I'm saying that if we want to really improve our health, we need to reestablish a connection with the life energy inside us. Then we will be able to support our health and healing—whether we see a doctor or not—by following the direction in which our chi wants us to go.

How does reconnecting with our chi inform and redirect our health? In many cases, it is subtle. People find that after they start to restore their chi through the practice of chi gung, t'ai chi, or Tao gung, old health problems they've carried around for years start to improve. It sort of sneaks up on them. They wake up one morning and realize that their knees aren't as stiff as they used to be or that they haven't needed an aspirin in weeks because their recurring headaches aren't recurring as often.

The health improvements people enjoy while restoring their chi are also sneaky, because the specific improvements may not happen in the order they predicted or wished. A woman who hopes t'ai chi will improve her sluggish digestion may find that her stomach problems don't get better right away, but surprisingly, her arthritis pain is almost gone. Or a man who never even considered t'ai chi or chi gung for physical health problems may come to our practice sessions hoping to relieve his intense job stress. After a few weeks, he is surprised to find that a long-standing back problem is getting better, even though his boss is still a tyrant.

The reason chi benefits are unpredictable is that chi has its own priorities and its own order of business. It will go where it sees the greatest need in our body or undertake what it considers the best first step in our body's repair. It won't necessarily go where we want it to go first.

Another way that the benefit of chi work can sneak up on people is when they gradually come to realize that they are automatically and effortlessly making better choices regarding their health. Their sensitivity to what their body needs gradually improves, and it slowly changes their behavior.

For example, after a period of weeks or months of consistent chi gung practice, people who smoke or overeat sometimes find that their desire for these habits gradually starts to drop away. They just don't like the way those old habits make them feel anymore. They feel like making better choices and find they suddenly have the willpower to do what they couldn't do before. Or their intuition may start to sense which foods are really bad for them and which foods energize them. Or they wake up one day and realize that they should look for a less stressful job, because they've learned to really enjoy the feeling of a calmer mind and don't want a job that hurts their health.

Why does this sensitivity or awareness of what their body needs improve? First of all, in the practice of chi gung moving meditation, we use *feeling* as we move. These folks have learned to really feel their bodies. They may never have experienced a solid connection to their own bodies before in their adult life. They've taken their bodies for granted. They may have spent years ignoring their "horses," beating and driving them too hard. Now that they can feel their bodies again, they really notice when their horses are tired, and they finally give them a much-needed rest. They feel that a certain food is upsetting their digestion or perhaps giving them a sluggish, weak feeling in their chi, so they stop eating that particular food. They realize that they feel ill at ease when their doctor doesn't listen to them carefully, so they decide to pick a new doctor whom they trust and who makes them feel more at ease.

It's truly amazing what just a few minutes a day of focusing your mind on the feeling in your body can do. In chi gung and t'ai chi practice, we work to fuse the mind, feeling, and chi back together. In our special practice, we try to move these elements of the self together as one whole, intact being. An infant's mind, feeling, life energy, and body all move together as one. Part of the damage we carry as adults is that we are split apart and disassociated from the many parts of ourselves. (How else could we drive a car while talking on the phone, eating a sandwich, and yelling at the kids in the backseat?)

That's another attribute that makes chi gung and t'ai chi different from Western or physical exercise. If you see joggers outside or people working out at a health club, they are often purposely distracting themselves by listening to loud music, talking to a friend, or watching a big-screen television. They want to occupy their minds with something else so they don't have to focus on the pain or exertion of their exercise, so the time passes faster, or perhaps because they want to multitask to save some time.

That type of distraction is the antithesis of chi gung. Our practice works to bring the scattered self into wholeness again. In moving meditation, the mind, feeling, chi, and body all move together. We focus our mind on that feeling, we move very slowly so we can savor and stay connected with the movement. Instead of letting any of our senses be entertained by outside stimuli, we focus each sense inward to detect and reconnect to that life energy.

Over time, we fuse all the many parts of ourselves back together, maybe for just a second at first, possibly a minute. But that fusion, no matter how brief, rebuilds and repairs the internal communication mechanism that is our birthright: this is the communication bridge that carries the messages between life energy, mind, and body. It's the real source of our good intuition and better choices. It's what we might call making the "chi connection." That connection allows our body to listen to the correct signal, or beneficial program, inside our chi.

When we don't have the chi connection, we are more prone to make harmful decisions or listen to bad advice. We are stuck with using our artificial thinking to make choices. Without the chi connection, we think artificial, processed food tastes good, and we prefer it. Or we don't even sense that we are overtired and try to function day in and day out with no sleep, relying on coffee and pills to keep us going. We pick activities and friends based on what will impress other people or what the newspaper tells us we should do, rather than choosing people and activities that *feel* good and right and true to us. Without the chi connection, these bad choices feel okay or even good to us because we are scattered and out of touch with our true feeling.

When you don't have the chi connection, your bad choices can divert, damage, and weaken your chi, causing you to make worse choices and leaving you with less energy to combat illness or repair injury. That damage leads to even more bad choices that hurt you even further, and your whole life can start to turn into a negative feedback loop of progressively draining choices and activities.

But if you make that chi connection, you make better choices, so your health improves. The more your health improves, the better your choices are and the more quickly you recover from illness and injury. This gives you more time and energy to keep practicing t'ai chi, which increases the strength of your chi connection, allowing you to have even more energy and make even better choices, and so on. You've thus created a new positive feedback loop for yourself.

Making the chi connection inside ourselves is the real goal of chi gung. Many people look for chi gung "shortcuts," and many books and teachers are happy to oblige them. What is a chi gung shortcut? It's when you have diabetes and look for a chi gung form specifically designed to regulate blood sugar. Or when you have a weight problem and seek a book of chi gung forms specifically designed to help you lose weight.

In one way, this is great, because through these shortcut methods, people may be exposed to chi gung for the first time and experience just a little of what working with their own life energy can do. On the other hand, those who practice this way can easily miss the real goal of chi gung and never experience its full range of benefits. If you simply do a handful of chi gung forms with the goal of losing weight, performing them like a physical exercise, you risk misunderstanding what it really means to make the chi connection. If you aren't working toward that connection, you will miss the best that chi gung has to offer.

That's why the practices in this book aren't targeted for bad knees, headaches, or diabetes. The chi gung practice I teach helps strengthen your chi in a comprehensive way and strengthen the connections between your chi and body, mind and body, mind and chi, and ultimately your chi and the Tao. When you approach chi gung in this traditional and authentic way, the way it was taught and preserved in the ancient Taoist temples, your potential gains are unlimited. Your chi is free not only to start working on your bad knees, diabetes, or weight problem, but to address hidden damage you may not even be aware of. Your chi connection can grow stronger and be there for you down the road to help with any unforeseen challenge in your life. Your true practice of chi gung can lift your physical condition and improve your mental and spiritual health.

MANY VOICES TELLING US WHAT TO DO

Stronger and cleaner chi lets you listen to that real voice inside that's trying to tell you to go in the right direction. Weak chi leaves you vulnerable to many confusing voices and to choosing the wrong one.

Not only are there confusing voices outside you—from the television, newspapers, and health businesses vying for your money—there are confusing voices *inside* your body as well, trying to tell you what to do. For example, you might have a bad program left over from old recycled energy that tells you to drink too much or take a lot of physical risks. That energy might steer you toward certain foods and activities that your body can't handle.

Even other life forms inside your body can tell you what to do. Am I getting this from a scary science fiction movie? Not at all. Did you know that more than two pounds of bacteria live inside the average adult? Scientists are finding that these bacteria can have a profound effect on your health and even send messages to your body that influence your moods and decisions.

The right or wrong bacteria in your body can make or break your immune system. They can improve or hinder the way you digest your food. While some bacteria can make you sick, many of them are necessary and beneficial to your health. You shouldn't assume you could even live without them.

What's even more interesting is that scientists are now finding that certain bacteria can send signals to your brain, guiding your cravings and behavior. For example, one study found that people who eat chocolate daily and have strong cravings for it have a certain strain of bacteria in their gut that is absent in those who don't like chocolate or who rarely eat it. Science is finding other correlations between food choices and the types of bacteria living inside you. When you really think about it, the question becomes, who is craving the chocolate? Are you choosing that chocolate bar from the real life energy inside you, or is there just a form of bacteria in your gut sending a chemical signal to your brain that screams, "Feed me chocolate!"

So we have advertisements and diet experts yelling, "Eat this, eat that"; recycled energy screaming, "I like this, I don't like that"; and bacteria demanding, "Feed me sugar/meat/chocolate now." It's no wonder we are confused. Those voices can drown out the real, true needs of our body, especially if our ability to make the chi connection is weak. If all those other voices are steering our decisions, our likes and dislikes, and overriding the better choices we should be making for our health, who is really in control? Who is the master?

If we want our true and original life energy back in control of our body, it is time to reconnect. To do that, we need to go inside and reconnect with our chi. We need to shut down the voices from outside and listen to the true voice within.

COMMUNICATING WITH OUR BODY AND CHI

How can we reestablish a connection with our chi? How can we learn to communicate with it?

First of all, we have to understand that this life energy signal is very subtle, very gentle. We have to be quiet and attentive to pick it up. We can't force it or demand that it make itself heard. If you want to see its gentleness, look at the life force in a new tree leaf unfurling in the spring, the patient work of a blade of grass making its way through a cement sidewalk, or the quiet building of an embryo growing into a fetus. We have to respect that subtlety. We can't connect if we go charging in with force to take control. No, it is a gentle and gradual process, like trying to match that gentleness and quietly approach the real feeling of ourselves deep inside, saying, "Self, I'm sorry I've ignored you for so long. Let's get acquainted with each other now. Let's try feeling. Let's be real. Let's work together."

Of course, this is only an illustration. We can't really *talk* to our body or life energy in the conventional sense. Why not? When we use human language, our body and life energy can't hear us. They can't understand our words. Life energy and the body are real. Language, thinking, and words are fake. They are made up in the mind for convenience. It would be wonderful if our body and chi could understand our language, because then we could just say, "Cancer, go away!" or "Craving for junk food, shut up!" or even "Cells, regenerate perfectly." Everyone could be healthy and live virtually forever.

I often stump my students by telling them they don't own their bodies: "You don't own your chi. Your chi owns you." After all, how can I really think that I own my body if I don't even know what any single cell in it is doing at any given time, much less tell that cell what to do? How in control am I if I can't consciously govern even the most minor symptoms of aging or illness? It's quite a stretch to think that I can talk to my body if I don't even own it.

If I want to tell my body what to do, it won't work. I must go to the master of this body, the owner, the one who can feel and know what each cell needs and influence what each cell does. If I can talk to the owner, then the owner can talk to my body. I need to build a relationship with that owner so I can tell the owner what I want my body to do. The master and owner of my body is that original life energy, the real me—not the ego or artificial mind that relies on thinking and language.

So how do we talk to our body's owner? How do we communicate with chi? We must use a medium and a language that our original life energy can understand. That language is *feeling*, because true feeling is very close to the frequency of life energy. Cells cannot understand brain waves and language. Feeling is a language much closer to that cellular language. That's why we always focus on feeling in moving meditation.

People often ask me, "Master, what should I eat? How should I exercise? How should I change my lifestyle?" As a master, I don't talk specifics about diet, exercise, and lifestyle in my books. I'd rather teach you how to use your sincere feeling to make your chi connection. If you reconnect with your chi with sincere feeling, your life energy will be able to tell you exactly what you should eat, how much you should exercise, and how you should live. Not only that, you can carry that ability to find your own answers with you for the rest of your life.

How can I write a book with specific advice about diet and lifestyle when everyone is different? If I write that everyone should eat three meals a day, what about a person with diabetes or hypoglycemia? Maybe her chi is telling her that she should be eating five times a day so her life energy can have the fuel it needs to restore balance and repair damaged cells inside her organs. Maybe somebody else's energy is desperately telling him to eat less often, maybe only two meals a day, so his digestive system or liver can have a rest. Both of these people are receiving the right and true message from their life energy at work inside them. If they follow my fake "expert" advice to eat three times a day, they might make a big mistake. That's why trying to find health advice in a book will always be limited and partial truth compared to reconnecting with your own chi.

When you make the chi connection and your chi says, "Eat more of *this*," it will no longer matter to you whether there are a thousand books that say *this* is bad for you. You will simply follow your chi. Even though everybody else is eating *that* and not *this,* you will ignore them. What difference does it make what everyone else is eating, if your energy is telling you what it needs and eating it makes you feel more balanced and alive? I repeat to my students over and over, "Go direct! Go connect!"

But initially, even what we feel as our gut or true feeling can lie to us because we have conditioned ourselves all our lives to want bad things. We get addicted to sugar, drugs, behaviors, artificial stimuli, and so forth. Through moving meditation, we not only reconnect to our true life energy feeling, but we clean up and purify that feeling so it begins to guide us toward what our life energy really needs rather than what it has been artificially conditioned to want. This restoration is a gradual process. Through moving meditation, we gradually clean up our energy layer by layer, until we get down to that original signal.

"But Master," you may say, "why should we ignore our own intelligence and the intelligence behind medical research that gives us advice on how to care for our health?" Don't ignore it. But realize there is another form of intelligence available to you, one that's constantly at work inside your body, and that it is much smarter than your brain or any university full of medical experts.

Do you know the moment a virus enters your body? No. When a virus first enters your body, you cannot feel it. Your mind doesn't consciously know it's there. You might not be aware of an invading virus until several hours after it's inside, when you start to get achy and tired and sport a fever. But there is a part of you that knows, that feels, and that starts to work right away. That's your chi. And if your chi is strong, it may take care of that virus so quickly that you will never know it was even there. Aren't you glad that your chi, not your brain, is in charge of monitoring the viral and other outside attacks to your body?

ORIENTAL MEDICINE, CHI, AND WAKING UP THE CELLS

The old Taoist masters understood the value of the chi connection. They knew that to heal the body, they must go through the chi. They were often asked to use their ability to work with life energy to heal others as well. That's how, over time, they evolved the many facets of Oriental medicine.

All the skills and arts they developed within this centuries-old medical system are primarily used to correct damage to and disharmony of the chi itself or to use chi as a medium to carry new messages to the cells and organ systems. They stumbled on ways to wake up that power and encourage it to flow the right way. Those methods used tools like needles and herbs to send messages through the chi to coax the repair of internal damage and imbalances. These ancient healing masters learned that even in cases of extreme organ failure, there were tricks they could use to extend life and give their patients a fighting chance.

You see, human organs are like construction sites. Did you ever drive by a new building or a road under construction? Did you notice that only some of the workers actually do the hard labor? The rest are hanging around—they're talking, drinking coffee, or taking a break. Day in and day out, the same hard-working guys are doing all the digging, pounding, and paving, while the other guys sit around. It doesn't seem fair, does it? Especially when you realize these same hard workers are the ones at highest risk for getting hurt on the job. If a big truck careens out of control through a road construction site, it's the hard workers in the middle of the road who will most likely get killed, not the guys sitting on the shoulder drinking coffee.

In your organs, certain cells are like those hard workers. They are in the front line, forced to detoxify the junk you eat, fight new infections, and digest your food. They're the ones that go to work first, stay busy longer, and do their jobs well. But the problem is that because they're the first ones to do their jobs, they are also the first to wear out or suffer damage. For example, if you accidentally eat some sort of poison, it's those hard-working cells that run to fight that poison first, neutralize it, and end up dying in the process.

But just like a construction site, your organs have many nonworkers too. You have billions of cells that have been placed on standby over time. It's as if those standby cells are playing cards in the back room, letting the hard workers take care of everything. In fact, those standby cells have become so lazy that they may have gone to sleep and forgotten how to wake up.

Somebody who has kidney failure or liver failure might really be in trouble and even face imminent death. What she doesn't know is that there may be millions of perfectly good cells still to be found in her kidney or liver. The trouble is that those cells don't know how to wake themselves up and do their job. They don't even know the hard workers have died and it's time for them to move into position and take over.

The old herbalists and healers found ways to send a message through the chi to say, "Wake up! Time to go to work!" They used herbs and acupuncture to stimulate the chi to coax those sleeping cells to do their job in hopes that it would buy them and their patients more time to effect a total cure.

This is one of many examples of how Oriental medicine can achieve results by working with chi. Unfortunately, most people seek out energy medicine only after a disease becomes acute or chronic. They don't even realize something's wrong until they are already in trouble. That's too bad, because if you wait until you have a disease before working to correct your chi, it takes much more time and energy to solve the problem. It's better to get rid of any imbalance before it progresses far enough to cause disease.

In the old days, the whole aim of a healer's work in Oriental medicine was to prevent disease before it could take hold. Making a commitment toward this same emphasis on prevention should be your approach to your own health.

The good news is that ongoing practice of t'ai chi moving meditation and chi gung exercises, like the ones you'll learn in this book, can gradually send a message through your chi to help restore, rebalance, and wake up those dormant cells before you ever reach the disease state. It can keep your chi resilient and strong so that ongoing repair in your body is done quickly and well, and your defenses against infection stay strong. It can correct small imbalances in your chi of which you might not even be aware. It can open up all those channels and meridians, flowing your life energy the right way so your health stays strong.

THE TAO FOLLOWS THE LAW OF NATURE

Another reason that we've lost our connection to our own chi is that we live unnatural lives. When we look back over human history, it's only in the last hundred years or so that we've had anything near the type of lifestyle we have today. For thousands upon thousands of years, humankind led much simpler lives. For the most part, we farmed or herded animals, living in small groups or family clans. We were close to the earth and much more in tune with the natural rhythms and seasons of nature and her cycles. We ate natural foods and enjoyed pure air and clean water.

Our bodies and life energy were never made to sit behind computers for hours every day, walled off from fresh air and sunshine, eating processed food out of a can, and driving home through noisy traffic to a twenty-story steel box in a crowded city. It's not that doing any of these things is wrong or that everyone should quit their jobs and move to the country immediately. It does mean that we need to be conscious of the fact that our bodies and our life energy are not accustomed to many of the unnatural, fast-paced, high-technology advancements with which we've surrounded ourselves. Our chi is under greater stress now, simply because it's trying to cope with our unnatural surroundings. Adapting to the fiercely unnatural lifestyle of today has cost us dearly in terms of chi. We need to do what we can to bring our original balance back.

Lao Tzu's *Tao Te Ching* says,

> In the universe, there are four great powers—and man is one of them. Man following the earth. The earth follows the heaven. And the heaven following the Tao. And the Tao following the Law of Nature.[1]

If even the Tao follows the law of nature, how can we hope to be healthy by going against it? Gradually allowing more space in your life for what is natural can go a long way toward helping you restore your chi connection. It doesn't require a sudden and dramatic lifestyle change. Bringing more natural elements into your daily routine can be as simple as walking outside for a few minutes during your lunch hour or opening a window at night and looking up at the stars for a few minutes before you retire. It may start with choosing fresh, natural fruits and vegetables instead of the type you buy in a can or cooking your own meal from whole foods rather than going to a fast-food drive-through. It may mean reducing harmful chemicals in your household or personal products.

Every small step you take to make your lifestyle more natural will help your chi connection. Why? Anything artificial and unnatural—including stale air, harmful toxins, and lifeless processed foods—can tax your chi. Every increment of chi that you use up to cope with all the fake, unnatural, harmful, or toxic elements in your life is that much less that you have to help you repair your internal organs, fight an infection, or quell a renegade cell that might be cancerous. On the positive side, every increment of chi that you free up by gradually building a more healthful and natural lifestyle is that much more that will be available for your body to use, repair, and guard itself.

Eventually, you'll also want as much chi as possible freed up in your life so you can do this chi gung work and restore that connection. Just as it is hard to have a conversation with someone who is frantically busy managing several crises at once, it is harder to connect with your chi if it is too busy managing multiple stressors from the unnatural assaults in your life. To make the chi connection, you need a calm place, a calm mind, and a lifestyle that supports your chi enough so that it is free to connect and communicate with you.

5

THREE LEVELS OF HEALING

WE ARE NOT one-dimensional people. We have many layers, many different aspects of ourselves, and many different frequencies of life energy. What are these different frequencies? Life energy can move very fast, or it can move more slowly.

When it moves slowly, it condenses and pulls in material to form your physical body. Think of the wide variety of physical tissues in your body. You have liquid tissues such as blood, digestive juices, and lymphatic fluid; you have soft, pliable tissues like muscle and tendons; and you have hard tissues like cartilage and bone. Despite the differences between these forms of body tissue, they are all alive. They all manifest a certain frequency of life energy to do their job. And although they are all alive, they are all also part of what we consider the physical dimension, representing a slower dimension of how life energy works.

Mind, thought, and chi flowing through your body are a faster form of life energy. These parts of you are moving so fast that they are invisible. And just as you have many different types of physical tissues, the chi or energy side of you can take on many forms. Consider the variety of moods, thoughts, and energy states you experience over the course of a few days. Your energy can change a lot, depending on the weather, the people you're involved with, your diet, or the variety of stressors in your life. The many different states of chi vary from person to person and from minute to minute. Chi is a finer, more subtle, higher frequency of life energy that has a profound influence on your mental state.

So we have the slower frequency of living physical tissue, the faster frequency of chi and the mind, and an even faster frequency of life energy that we might refer to as spiritual energy. This would include your Te as well as energy imprints or coatings surrounding it that operate beyond the physical, energy, and thought dimensions. You can even have bits of negative spiritual energy following you around—what other religions call karma, debt, or even sin. Spiritual energy is higher in power and frequency than what we call the chi or mental level, and it is much higher than the physical dimension. Because it operates at such a faster and higher frequency, it is even more subtle and harder for us to detect.

All three dimensions of ourselves—the physical level, the chi or mental level, and the spiritual level—interact and affect each other. That's why it is important to keep each level in good shape in order to enjoy physical health as well as mental and spiritual well-being. If any one of these three levels has a problem, or if you violate any laws governing any of these three dimensions, there can be a penalty or a negative impact on your life.

TO FIX A PROBLEM, GO TO THE LEVEL OF ITS CAUSE

Most of the best physicians understand the following basic law of healing: to bring about a cure, you must go to the root or cause of the problem, not simply treat the symptoms. Let's illustrate how this law works. If you go to the doctor with recurring headaches, a mediocre practitioner will simply give you some aspirin and send you on your way. A true physician will do much more. She'll take the time to ask you about what's going on in your life, what you're eating, and if you have had any recent injuries or stress that could be causing your headaches. She will do a physical exam to see if you have any hidden health issues that could be contributing to the problem and try to pinpoint and eliminate whatever it is that is causing your headaches. She will go to the root cause in an effort to bring about real healing, not just give you medication to treat your symptoms.

In our examination of how to restore our life energy, we are going to take that same law and apply it on an even higher level. We are going to restate the law this way: to bring about a cure, you must go to the energy level where the cause of the problem resides. When you have a problem in your life, be it a health problem or any other life problem, the *source* of that problem could be in the physical dimension, the mental or chi dimension, or the spiritual dimension. If you don't treat the problem at the level where it has its source, you won't have lasting success.

Let's take a look at how this might apply to a health problem. Your condition could have a physical cause, or it could have what we call a chi (the energy or mental level) cause; it might even have a root cause at the spiritual level. To solve that problem, no matter what it is, you need to fix it at the same level as the root cause. The cause of a problem—be it in the physical, chi, or spiritual dimension—is usually a result of a violation of laws governing that particular dimension.

If the cause of your illness is at the physical level, that may be fairly easy to fix. You can go ahead and use conventional remedies. They will probably work just fine. Let's say you scraped your elbow after falling off your bicycle. It's effective to treat the scrape at the physical level by washing it off and applying a bandage. You can also prevent further scrapes by tightening the loose bolt on the front wheel of your bike or simply taking curves a little slower next time. These are all physical measures taken to treat an injury caused in the physical dimension or to eliminate the violation of physical laws (laws such as "Bicycles become unstable when they have loose wheels and turn corners too quickly").

Most of what we consider conventional medicine works at the physical level of illness. Diet, pills, bandages, surgery, vitamins, massage, manipulation, and so on—all of these are concrete physical ways to deal with physical problems. Even molecular medicine and energy therapies such as ultrasound and radiation happen in the physical dimension and are meant to affect you in a purely physical way.

Let's say you have heartburn every time you eat spicy food. You go to the doctor, and she tells you that you should stop eating spicy food. You do, and your heartburn goes away. Or maybe you still get heartburn, and your doctor prescribes an antacid; after taking the pills, your heartburn goes away. This is another example of a health problem that had a physical cause and was cured by physical means.

What if diet changes and antacid don't work? You've tried everything you can on the physical level, but you still get heartburn. Chances are the root of your problem is at a higher level, perhaps it is an energy problem. Your chi flow may be blocked, weak, excessive, or carrying the wrong signal to your internal organs.

Healing at this level is different. It works directly with the chi to eliminate the energy imbalance or impure energy signal that is causing the problem.

We previously mentioned that almost all Oriental medicine works in this way. While on the outside it may look like acupuncture and herbs are physical tools, they are designed to remedy a chi problem by changing the way your energy flows. Thus, Oriental medicine is founded on a completely different philosophy than Western medicine.

So when you go to an Oriental medicine practitioner, he will try to diagnose whether the chi flowing to your stomach is too weak to fuel good digestion, the upward flow of chi in your body is too excessive, or the energy condition of any other organ systems are contributing to your heartburn.

An *energy healer,* or someone who can flow energy to you through his hands, will do the same thing. He will use his energy to try to change your chi flow and bring it back into balance once again.

The range in skill between one acupuncturist and another, one energy healer and the next, can be vast. For example, some acupuncturists are like that mediocre doctor who simply gives you an aspirin for your headache. They take your symptom and consult a book that tells them where to put needles for a headache, which herbs fix indigestion, or what acupuncture point might relieve a cough. Yes, their treatment may work sometimes, but it's a lower level of energy medicine performed without a full understanding of the practice's potential.

A superior acupuncturist will go much deeper. He will examine your tongue, your fingernails, your eyes, your diet, and various pulses in your body, and he will work toward an individualized diagnosis of your personal energy condition. Only then will he carefully consider which treatments to use. He uses a higher wisdom in trying to evaluate and work with your specific energy pattern.

An even higher level of energy healer, one that you will rarely find anymore, is one who has worked many years to establish his own chi connection. He has learned to be able to listen to and communicate with his own chi. Then, because he is so sensitive to his own chi, when he takes your pulse or places a needle in a point on your body, he can actually feel and communicate with your chi. He uses *his* chi connection to pick up signals and information from *your* chi and get a much clearer picture of what's going on inside your body. In the old days, such healers could even send their chi signal into your body in an effort to reprogram your life energy. They would send their chi through a needle with a message such as, "Speed up," or "Slow down," or "Go here," or "Go there." They would infuse your energy with their dominant, healthier program, which would bring your internal energy system into balance. This took a lot of practice, and sending such an energy signal into a patient could tax a healer's personal energy. They learned how to do chi gung, t'ai chi, and Tao gung so they could recharge and strengthen themselves, as well as protect themselves from any damage to their chi that might occur from connecting to the energies of their sick patients.

But let's go back to your heartburn. Let's say you've tried acupuncture and herbs and have even seen a really good energy healer whom your friend recommended, but your heartburn keeps coming back after a few days or weeks. No amount of physical-level or even energy-level work appears to help.

Such stubborn problems sometimes have a spiritual cause. This is that karma, debt, or sin that most religions refer to time and again. The violation may be something you did when you were younger or something you're doing wrong right now. It may even be a violation attached to that recycled energy you picked up when you came into this life.

Spiritual-level problems are tricky because we can't easily see or understand what the cause is. The frequency of the spiritual level is so high that we can't tune in to it. We need help from somebody who can see and reach that dimension of spiritual energy.

Many ancient temples had special monks who were trained to see into and communicate with spiritual dimensions. When these monks connected with that highly refined frequency of the spiritual level, they could help people by telling them what caused their problem and by negotiating a solution or forgiveness of that problem at the spiritual level.

Very few individuals have that ability today. Many claim to have spiritual powers or gifts, but these are often lower level or even artificial tricks. If you are lucky enough to meet a real monk with such abilities, you are fortunate indeed.

You can also see echoes and remnants of this spiritual ability in some of the religious rites that have carried over to today. Many of the rituals a priest or minister or rabbi performs in a weekly worship service or in various consecration or sacramental activities are based on ancient energy practices designed to connect and communicate with that spiritual dimension. The relentless passage of time, however, has generally left only the shell of the ritual behind. Few modern-day religious leaders actually practice rituals with the potent ability to connect with spiritual energy. The rituals simply remain as reminders to point you in the direction of the spiritual world to look for answers. They bear witness that, for centuries, humankind has sensed that there are spiritual sources and spiritual answers for many of its problems.

The reality that the spiritual level can affect our health is evidenced by newly documented results of the effectiveness of prayer in healing. Researchers found that when they monitored results for a large group of people, when everything else was equal, sick people had a slight advantage in recovery if they had people who prayed for them. Even when we lack the training of the old monks, if we pray with sincerity and a pure heart, we can sometimes reach that pure, clear frequency of the spiritual world without even knowing it.

THE RELATIONSHIP BETWEEN THE THREE LEVELS

What you need to know is that there is a hierarchical relationship between the physical, chi, and spiritual levels. Higher-frequency energy always dominates with respect to lower-frequency energy. The spiritual level is higher than and can set limits on or control what happens on the chi level. The chi level is higher than and can set limits or control what happens on the physical level.

What does this mean to you? To solve a problem, you have to fix that problem on the same level as its cause, *or* you must go to an even higher level. Lower-level solutions won't work.

If you have a health problem that's caused by a violation at the chi level, no amount of physical help will cure it. You can eat the healthiest food, see the best doctors, take the right medicines, and do everything perfectly, but you will not be able to correct your problem because the physical level is lower than the cause of that problem.

If your problem is rooted in the spiritual level, no amount of physical medicine or chi healing will help. You can see an acupuncturist or an energy healer, eat right, exercise, and spend all day at the doctor's office, but nothing will work. Why? Because both physical- and energy-level solutions are at a lower level than the spiritual cause of your problem. For spiritual problems, you need spiritual remedies.

You have to meet each problem at the level of its cause or else you must find a way to go higher. This rule explains why going to the doctor or seeking energy healing doesn't always work or works differently from one person to the next. You've seen it before: some people can strive seemingly forever with the same nagging illness. If your headache is caused by a chi imbalance in your liver, you can take aspirin every day but it won't stop your recurring headaches. It would be like firefighters showing up to put out a house on fire. They can bring out all their hoses and work all day and all night. They might reduce the flames somewhat. But if they don't know that what's really causing the fire is a broken gas pipe in the basement, that fire is going to keep burning and relighting itself until the gas is shut off.

This rule not only applies to problems of health, it applies to recurring problems in our lives as well. It applies to marital problems, social problems, financial problems, and personal issues in much the same way that it applies to health. Life problems can also have their cause in the physical, chi, or spiritual level. To solve any problem in life, you must resolve it at the level of its cause.

Knowing the relationship between these three levels can be to your advantage. If you go to a level higher than your problem, you can easily manage everything happening on lower levels. If you are able to connect to, strengthen, and purify your chi, you will have a much easier time dealing with your physical health problems. You'll also have an easier time dealing with the mundane stresses of daily life. Likewise, if you can strengthen and purify your energy to the degree that you can understand, communicate with, and reconcile yourself with that spiritual dimension, the power will automatically adjust and flow down to the chi and physical levels. Your energy will automatically become stronger and flow where and how it should, and your physical troubles, as well as stubborn obstacles in your life, will melt like ice on a warm day.

Of course, the best approach when you have a serious health problem is to work on all three levels at the same time. If you have life-threatening cancer, you might not have time to figure out what the cause is. You don't have the luxury of time to do detective work, build a chi connection from scratch, or let chi gung alone help repair your body. You have to mount a full-scale attack. You need to find physical-, energy-, and spiritual-level help as best you can—right away! So if you are enjoying relatively good health as you read this book, don't wait to make your chi connection. If you wait until you are too sick or too old, you may not have the luxury of time you have now.

THERE ARE NO SHORTCUTS

We talk about the three layers—physical, chi, and spiritual—as if they were separate phenomena, but that is just for the purposes of study and explanation. Actually, at their root, they are all part of the one overarching energy of the Tao. Everything originates from the same Source, and each level is interconnected with and continually affecting the others. Again, they are merely the same energy operating at different frequencies, just as water is water, even though it may take the form of ice, liquid, or steam, depending on at what frequency or speed those water molecules are moving.

This interconnection between the physical, chi, and spiritual levels is why chi gung is so important. You see, chi gung moving meditation can work on all three levels, because it helps raise the speed and frequency of your overall energy.

By fusing your mind back to the feeling in your physical body and fusing both back to the sensation of your chi, every part of you benefits. You bring those parts back into better harmony with each other. They start to vibrate in tune with each other again. Spending time in moving meditation raises the connection level between body and mind, body and chi, mind and chi, chi and spirit, and mind and spirit. Again, you are bringing these scattered parts of yourself back toward the original holistic function they were meant to have.

That natural harmony between mind, body, and spirit needs repair because we spend most of each day connecting to very low-level frequencies. If I read the newspaper or watch television, I am connecting to a low level of input. But if I connect my mind to the feeling of life energy within my body, and I move and flow with that feeling, I connect to a higher level. The purer I get, the higher the level I can connect to within myself, eventually connecting to the spiritual level. The gradual improvement in this connection filters through progressively higher levels of energy and programming to my spirit, mind, and body.

That is why the old Taoist monks spent so much of their lives in meditation and chi gung practice. They knew that if we are sincere and pure, this way of living can raise our energy level high enough to restore harmony even at the spiritual level of our being.

Some people will read this chapter and decide to run out and find an energy healer or an acupuncturist, or maybe they'll be lucky enough to find an authentic spiritual reader or healer. After all, it seems like an easy shortcut. Why not take a few herbs to balance my chi or have someone flow her energy through her hands to correct my life energy signal? Why should I take the long road of investing in building my own chi connection when I can get a boost from outside? Some people even call or write to me and ask, "Master, can you send me your chi and heal me?"

Here are the words such people may not want to hear: there are no shortcuts. Yes, Oriental medicine can work wonders with correcting a chi problem. Sure, there are healers and masters who can send you their chi to strengthen your energy and help your chi flow the right way. Yes, there are spiritual monks and masters who can see and even help you rectify a spiritual problem through prayer.

However, once that outside source fixes you and you return to your same old thoughts, habits, lifestyle—the same body with the same recycled energy you started with—how long will that healing last? How long will the energy charge, chi correction, or spiritual correction last? Not very long. Within days, weeks, months, or a year, that old faulty energy pattern will likely return like a bad habit. You'll fall back into your old programming. Your original problems will come back, or you will pick up a new problem somewhere else.

If you receive a temporary boost to your energy from an outside source, it can feel terrific. It's as if someone lifted you in a helicopter and placed you on a mountaintop. The trouble is that if someone else puts you on that mountaintop, the first strong wind can blow you right down.

But if you use chi gung, t'ai chi, and Tao gung on a regular basis and win back your own pure energy signal, it means you've climbed the mountain by yourself. That gain becomes yours for far longer. You've earned the chi connection, and nobody can take it away. It will be much harder to knock you off that mountaintop. Also, if you've built your chi connection, when and if you do feel the need to resort to outside healing or spiritual help, you can hold on to its benefits much longer.

6

MOVING MEDITATION IS THE KEY

WHAT IS THE MOST important attribute of chi gung? What is the key element shared by chi gung, t'ai chi, and Tao gung? Why are these three practices considered different and placed in a separate category from other meditation systems? The answer is that they all rely on *moving meditation*.

Chi is our life energy, and that energy is created and supported by the piece of God's energy inside us, our Te. Remember that life energy is alive, and living things move. Everything in the universe is made of God's energy, and God's energy is alive. That's why everything in the universe is always in motion.

On the smallest scales, the molecular, atomic, and subatomic levels, everything is always in motion. To my knowledge, no physicist has yet been able to find a submolecular or subatomic particle that remains perfectly still. They all move.

On the largest scales, the earth always spins on its axis and around the sun, our galaxy spirals, and even the universe itself rotates and expands.

To be in motion is to be in harmony with the universe, because the universe is always in motion. To be in motion is to be in harmony with life energy, because life energy is always in motion. To be in motion is to be in harmony with God's energy, because God's energy is always in motion. Movement is life, while stillness is death and decay.

This is why moving meditation is our main pathway back to restoring our connection to our true life energy. We want to be in the closest harmony to the original nature of life energy, and part of that original nature is motion.

Most other meditation traditions require sitting and seeking stillness. But stillness is an illusion. Look around—nothing is ever truly still. Even if you were sitting in meditation, still like a statue and your mind profoundly calm, your cells would still be in active motion, busy absorbing nutrients and cleansing waste matter. Your blood would still be coursing through your veins. You would still be breathing in and out.

Stillness is an ego-created idea. It is not the nature of life and the universe. In reality, everything moves. If everything moves and I insist on not moving, then I am automatically in conflict with the universe. If the universe is always moving, then I want to flow with it in order to be in harmony with and connect to it.

This is why, of all the ancient wisdom traditions, chi gung, t'ai chi, and Tao gung are so powerful. They comprise the only system that preserves the wisdom of moving meditation. Through moving meditation, we can actually get closer to matching the energy frequency of the universe and make the connection with the source of all energy—the Tao.

There is a place for sitting meditation. However, true sitting meditation is not for sitting still and doing nothing. While you are sitting and meditating, you still have to concentrate on the energy flow inside. If you are not feeling and flowing your energy during your sitting meditation, then you are just thinking. Thinking only takes you through that labyrinth of artificial imaginings in your head.

In the oldest forms of Zen, Buddhist, and Taoist meditation, sitting meditation also included internal circulation. Many of the sitting meditation masters were circulating life energy inside themselves. They were moving their concentration inside, thinking about flow and ultimately feeling that flow. On a beginner's level, even what might be termed "still meditation" becomes moving meditation when you feel and follow your breath as it expands in and out. Sitting meditation that follows the natural breath as it moves can be very fruitful because it is a sitting version of moving meditation.

I often tell my students this simple truth, "In order to grow, you must flow." You simply cannot grow, strengthen, and purify your chi without feeling, flowing, and moving it. That's why meditation is only part of the answer. You also have to move!

Just as meditation without movement is only half of the equation, physical movement without meditation is only half. Perform chi gung or t'ai chi as if it were merely a slow form of physical exercise and you'll miss the best part. You have to add in focused, sincere meditation for that movement to strengthen your chi.

Move and meditate, meditate and move. You cannot separate the two if you want to work with your chi. Moving is wrong, meditation is wrong—it must be both. Like two sides of the same coin, they must be fused together to be worth something. If I cut a quarter in half lengthwise and give you both pieces, it doesn't have any value. Cut in half, the coin is worth nothing.

Thinking about swimming and actually swimming in the water are two different things. They must be combined. If I just sit and think about swimming, what good does that do? Conversely, if somebody pushes me into the water while I'm *not* thinking about swimming but engrossed in my daydreams, I may flounder, splash, and swallow a few mouthfuls of water before I can figure out what to do. To swim successfully, I must combine the two. I must think about swimming and then get into the water and move.

Treat moving meditation like one inseparable event. Treat it like one word, *movingmeditation,* and you'll have the right idea. When moving combines with meditation, it matches up with the facts and the truth of the Tao. The original all-encompassing One Energy of the Universe is both "everywhere and always conscious" and "everywhere and always in motion." It is never one without the other. It is always meditating and always moving.

CALMING THE MIND

All forms of meditation attempt to calm the mind. It's usually a vain attempt because if you meditate, you'll soon find that it's very hard to stop the mind from wandering around. As I said before, stillness is an illusion. In meditation, we prove it to ourselves, since we cannot even achieve stillness inside our own mind.

The mind was made to think. It continues to think and chatter, even when we wish it would stop during our practice. Even in our sleep, it is still going, going, going. Rather than fight with the mind and try to force it into stillness, in our moving meditation practice, we cooperate with it instead. We recognize that the mind needs to be busy, so we give it something productive to do. We set it to work trying to feel the life energy inside us and the center of the lower stomach.

It's like the old analogy says, "The mind is like a monkey." You cannot stop a monkey from jumping and climbing around and getting into trouble. That's its nature. But if you give the monkey something to do, like peel a banana, it will calm down and focus. In moving meditation, we give the monkeylike mind something concrete to do so we can stay focused and calm. We throw it a banana by telling it to feel and focus on the lower stomach and/or feel our life energy as we move. If our monkey jumps away, we gently bring it back to its task. No need to try to change the monkey's nature or fight with it. We train the monkey to work for us, not against us.

Bringing the mind gently back to the feeling inside the body, especially to the lower stomach, is the heart of moving meditation. It is the heart of restoring our chi. Why? Because we bring all of that chi that thinking normally disperses, grab it, and channel it back into our body, sending it back to its source.

Think of your body as a candle and your mind as the flame. The flame sends light and heat out and away from itself. It's beautiful. However, that flame burns up fuel as it literally eats up the candle, and the candle's life gets shorter and shorter.

In moving meditation, we reverse this process. It's as if we somehow take all the energy from the candle flame, and instead of letting it burn away, we turn it inward and condense and focus it in such a way that it can help feed, build up, and maintain the candle. Then the candle will not melt as fast as it used to. This can happen by channeling the energy of the mind back into the feeling of energy inside our body. We recapture energy that would otherwise have been burned up and lost in the ether of thinking. We create a closed-circuit system.

That's also why some of the old Taoist and Buddhist teachings call the mind the "flower." Life energy is considered the root. A flower is so flamboyant and colorful, but it is a display that will soon wither and die. A root sits there quietly, but it is powerful and stable. The root is the life source of nourishment and life for the flower. So to tap into that resilient, strong, nourishing power, we have to rejoin the flower of the mind with its root.

FOCUSING ON THE LOWER STOMACH

One of the jobs we give our mind during chi gung practice is to focus inside on the center of our lower stomach. The Taoist masters call this spot the *tan tien* or *dan tian*. We want our mind to focus on that area because this is an important part of going backward.

Remember that our goal is to go backward so we can wake up the original power from when we were just a single cell. From what location did that single cell begin its journey? From where did it connect and receive nourishment from our mother? From the center of the lower stomach, through the umbilical cord.

When you were an embryo, you were curled up in your mother's lower stomach. Her womb was the cradle of life for you. Your nourishment came into your own lower stomach through the umbilical cord. Your body curved and formed itself around this spot, which is the home of original life energy's first entry into the human world. It's your original home. That is why our practice always returns there to look for the original energy signal. We return to the tan tien to wake up that memory. We go backward and return home.

You'll find that, later in the book, most of the moving meditation exercises to restore chi urge you to relax, keep a calm mind, and begin each exercise with your hands in front of your tan tien, or navel area. We use this training to try to bring up the old memory of how we were when we were an embryo or a single cell. This is why we also bring our hands back to our tan tien at the close of every moving meditation. We keep reminding our energy to return home.

MOVING LIKE A SINGLE CELL

With most reputable t'ai chi and chi gung instructors, the first pieces of advice you'll hear as a beginner are to stay relaxed and to keep your body curved and your form round. The movements of t'ai chi and chi gung moving meditation have no jagged movements and no hard angles. The movements are round and follow a natural curve. Why? The universe is round, the galaxy is round, stars are round, planets are round, a single cell is round. We want to harmonize with that powerful universal energy, so we make ourselves and our motions round.

Simple tips like these are actually very important, because following them will encourage your chi to flow the right way. This is because a rounded form is more like how you were when you were a single cell developing into an embryo in your mother's womb.

Then you were round and soft, almost fluid. You floated quietly in a world of liquid, very relaxed. There were no hard angles or lines. As an embryo, all of your parts and limbs started as small nubs, almost spherical, while your developing body curved in on itself naturally. Your body developed according to the natural way your life energy flowed. By thinking of that embryo, you can see that your life energy originally flowed in natural curves, creating your body section by rounded section.

We mimic those natural, relaxed curves in moving meditation. For example, we keep our elbows neither bent nor straight, but gently curved. We keep our wrists neither bent nor straight, but gently curved. Today, we can use a thin, fiber-optic cable to take pictures of a living embryo as it develops into a fetus; we will find that the embryo's elbows and wrists are soft and gently curved, the same way we hold them in our practice.

By mimicking the way our single cell and embryo moved and flowed as closely as possible in our moving meditation, we have a better chance of waking up that memory.

MOVING TOGETHER AS ONE PIECE

A single cell is one whole being. It functions as one piece. When it flows, everything flows. The substance, intelligence, and energy of that cell all flow together as one. They are not separate, they are fused together, intact.

That's why, in moving meditation, we want to practice so that when we move, everything moves together. When we move up, our mind thinks up, we feel our energy and let it move up, our body follows that feeling of energy and moves up, and we inhale and expand up—all at the same time. We want to feel as if each part of our body is connected to every other part. Everything is moving together, or up, at the same time. Again, we want to mimic as closely as possible the condition of that original single cell.

Right now, we just practice this. But as time goes on, the fusion becomes real. Someday, when we think "left," our life energy will automatically flow left, our body will naturally follow it and move left, and we will effortlessly move left as one piece. When we do that, we're flowing like our single cell!

We want to fuse all of these elements back into one so our energy remembers what it's like to be intact. If it can fuse together and stay intact, it has a chance to pick up that original signal. As adults, we cannot stay intact twenty-four hours a day, but at least we do it for five minutes here and there. That's why you do chi gung—you start to bring yourself back and stay intact just long enough to remind your energy of its original way. This gives your system a chance to restore itself. Your immune system, your breathing, everything starts to remember that original energy and how you should be.

We don't "learn" or teach ourselves chi gung or t'ai chi, we merely use it to remind our body of the original way it used to move. In our practice, it's as if we tell our body, "That's how you moved before. C'mon, let's go. You know how to move that way."

In your mother's womb, you moved like we do in chi gung but you lost this natural way because you became "smarter." You got an artificial education not only in how to think, but also in how you should move. You learned how you were supposed to move in order to hold a pencil or ride a bike, and you thought you were getting better and better, smarter and smarter. Not exactly. By learning artificial, rigid, and mechanical ways of moving, you were just giving up all the power and potential of the natural motion of flow you had before.

THE POWER OF WEAKNESS

The only way you are going to trigger life energy is when mind, body, and breathing all fuse together. But as they fuse and move together, you must remain very relaxed, gentle, and weak.

Is a baby physically strong and aggressive in the mother's womb? No, it is very weak. But does that mean the baby has no power? Absolutely not. In weakness lies great power, because a baby is relaxed enough to pick up and use the original energy signal.

Likewise, we cannot pick up and use that original energy signal unless we are weak. Does *weak* mean limp and passive? No. *Weak* means not relying on our own strength and power. We stay relaxed and alert, looking for that subtle sensation, that signal, not relying on conventional physical force. The more we rely on our own power and strength, the more we shut off that subtle, weak signal of original energy.

Although it is hard to detect at first, that weak signal is very powerful. How powerful can it be? Because an embryo is still pure enough to use the weak power in the mother's womb, that embryo is the boss. It sends out a signal to tell the mother what to do. If it needs calcium and doesn't get it, it will pull the calcium straight out of its mother's bones if necessary. If it needs a certain vitamin or a particular mineral, the mother will crave specific foods that provide exactly what it needs. Does that embryo in the womb accomplish this by talking, pushing, or moving around? No. It's just floating in there. It takes control by sending its message via that subtle but powerful life energy signal.

When a baby is born, does a baby crawl and pull his way out of the womb? No. He sends a signal to tell his mother's body to secrete the hormone to cause uterine contractions. He doesn't secrete anything, just sends a signal that sets labor in motion.

The mother and her body have to obey this signal. Why? Because the baby's energy is new, closer to that original source of life energy, so his signal is more powerful. Whether the mother is eighteen, twenty-eight, or thirty-eight years old, she is more polluted, disconnected from, and further away from the original source than her baby is. She can no longer connect to her life energy signal in the same way that her baby can. Because the baby's energy is closer to the original source, the signal he can radiate is dominant. That's how this "weak" force works. And once that weak little baby comes, watch out! Pretty soon the whole world revolves around him. Just ask his parents who wears out whom.

Lao Tzu asks in the *Tao Te Ching,* "Can you be like a baby?" He goes on to teach that this is an important component of achieving the Tao. The question doesn't imply that you should look like a baby. It means that you need to feel and follow your internal energy like a baby, tapping into that weak power.

A newborn's bones are weak, his muscles soft, but his grip is firm.

He has no experience of the union of man and woman, but his sexual energy is whole. It is because his life energy is full and strong.

He could cry all day without becoming hoarse. It is because he is in perfect harmony."[1]

Babies are whole and spontaneously one with their chi inside. They are not strong in the conventional way we define strength, but like Lao Tzu says, let a baby grab your finger. It is very hard to pry off her clutch because her whole being—mind, feeling, energy, the whole body—is fused and focused on the feeling of holding your finger.

It's because we want to tap into this same power that relaxation is a primary principle of chi gung and moving meditation. Whenever you tense up, the first thing to suffer is the sensation and feeling of your chi. If you're strong and stiff, then of course you won't be able to feel that weak, subtle signal. If your body tenses up, then your chi won't be able to flow properly. You won't be able to practice cooperating with it and using it to propel your body. Then your chi won't be able to grow strong.

Relaxation is the core of chi gung and t'ai chi, because your body's physical strength and chi compete against each other, canceling each other out. That's why you try to relax. You don't want your muscles to be dominant in comparison with your chi. It's precisely because you have spent most of your life moving with tension that your chi is now lagging behind. Relaxing gives it the chance to catch up. Gentle and easy, never using any strenuous motion—this is the right way to practice your chi gung. Anytime you are struggling, strained, or tense, your life energy shuts off and doesn't want to flow.

Some people take the wrong approach to moving meditation and say, "Oh, let's put some weights on our arms and get stronger while we do chi gung." No! Then you are going in the opposite direction, because you'll focus on your muscles. You'll create more tension, rely on mechanical motion, and ignore your signal, your feeling. If you try to increase your physical strength, you may get stronger and more toned, but you'll never learn to depend on that feeling. You won't give your life energy—that rich, sensitive, and subtle signal—a chance to grow.

THE POWER OF FLOW

When we want to strengthen our muscles, we can use physical exercise. When we want to strengthen our energy, we must use flow, because that is how energy naturally travels in the universe.

Moving by flow is actually more powerful than mechanical motion that jumps from here to there. Think of what happens when an earthquake is followed by a tsunami. That tremendous energy in the earth is displaced through the water, which carries it through flow across an entire ocean with incredible destructive force. Water is soft, but it harnesses the power of flow to carry that energy. You don't scoop up all the water from one part of the ocean and dump it in another part to cause that effect. The power is in the flow.

Flow is also how a single cell moves. When you were a single cell, you didn't jump from here to there; even when you split into new cells, you did everything through flow. Nourishment flowed in and waste products flowed out through your cell walls. Anything happening inside that cell happened through flow. A single cell doesn't have arms or legs, but it can flow to expand or contract, cave in or bulge out in one spot, and thereby move itself around. It flows all of its substance inside itself and also flows with what surrounds it. That's why in t'ai chi moving meditation, we learn to flow that feeling of life energy inside us and to flow with everything happening outside us.

A single cell doesn't think, doesn't visualize, doesn't imagine. It flows and lets life energy propel everything. In t'ai chi moving meditation, we don't rely on just thinking or imagining that we are flowing, we really let our energy flow and learn to let that flow propel our body. We may use thought and imagination to get our practice going, but at some point, we trade them for real feeling and real flow.

How important is flow? If our energy doesn't flow, we die. If the energy flow inside our body slows down, we age. If it is interrupted in any way, we get sick. I'm not talking about blood circulation. I'm talking about the integrity of our life energy's flow, the same power that causes our cells to split and every individual cell to work together to maintain the integrity of our whole being to give us the power to think, move, pray, feel, and exist.

Harnessing the power of that flow is central to restoring our life energy. We need to flow if we want to clean and purify all the junk that's attached to our chi. To purify dirty water, the water must flow through a filter at some point. We filter our chi by first calming and settling our mind, getting rid of all the junk in our thinking, and then flowing our chi. A calm mind focused on feeling is like a filter for our flowing energy.

We flow and practice until our mind wanders and tries to interrupt us again. We don't stop; we simply calm our mind again, focus on our feeling, and flow some more. Through this practice, we gradually increase our sense of feeling and awareness throughout our body.

Learning new chi gung forms is valuable to a point, but it can never replace learning just one or two forms and practicing them sincerely with flow. We don't learn new forms to collect them and show off. They are valuable simply because they help us learn how to flow our energy in several different directions, flushing out stagnant areas and bringing clean life energy to every hidden corner of ourselves.

Your goal in chi gung practice is literally to change your life energy. That real change is what delivers all the benefits of chi gung practice. But the benefits will only come from flow, not from the physical exercise alone. It's the flow of the energy that changes you.

You just practice, relax, and let your energy flow. You subject yourself to that flow. It's like when you subject yourself to the sunshine because you want to get a suntan. You don't have to do anything special. You just subject yourself to being outside in the sunshine. Give yourself over to the revitalizing message of moving meditation by being in and subjecting yourself to the flow. When you do chi gung with feeling and flow, staying relaxed and calm, the changes happen automatically.

MOVE YOUR ENERGY, NOT JUST YOUR BODY

Our day-to-day movements are very mechanical. Over time, we've laid down the hardwiring inside our body so that our brain can tell our hands, arms, legs, back, and muscles to do exactly what it wants. We are very good at this. We are quite "handy," in that we can clap, dance, twiddle our thumbs. Our brain-to-muscle coordination is so good that we can ride a bicycle, run up and down stairs, and rub our bellies and pat our heads at the same time.

In fact, we are so good at direct mechanical motion that we don't even have to concentrate on our movements; we do them automatically, almost unconsciously. Our brain says, "Pick up pencil," and our hand automatically reaches over to pick up a pencil, even while we are concentrating on something else. Perhaps you have driven to the store, preoccupied by something else, and wondered how you got there. Your mechanical motion is so automatic, so ingrained, that your brain and muscles can work by themselves with little concentration or effort from you.

The communication circuit for direct mechanical motion is simple:

Brain → Muscles = Movement

In moving meditation, we work to rediscover and reprogram a different communication path inside ourselves. We relearn an *indirect* form of motion that relies on chi. During chi gung practice, instead of our brain telling our muscles to move, we use it to tell our chi—the feeling of life energy—to move, and that feeling moves our body:

Brain → Feeling/Chi → Body = Movement

This difference is important. Moving by feeling is actually how your body was originally designed to move. It's a far better and easier way.

As an example of this difference, imagine a primitive car in which you must stick your foot out of a hole in the floor and push against the pavement to stop. That is direct: your brain tells your foot to push and stop the car. This is just like your body's form of mechanical motion.

But if you have a more advanced car, you have a hydraulic braking system. When you want to stop, your mind tells your foot to push the brake pedal, which sends a message through the system, and it's that system that puts pressure on the braking mechanism to stop the car. Far more efficient and effective, this is a parallel to what we are trying to achieve in the indirect motion of chi gung. We don't just use our brain to tell our body to move. It is our meditation that moves our energy, and in turn, our energy moves our body.

So after you learn the physical motions of a few chi gung exercises in Chapter 7, start focusing more on the feeling of life energy inside you. You will gradually learn to move that feeling, that energy.

It will feel awkward at first. It's hard to concentrate and move your feeling rather than just your muscles. Your feeling of chi may be nonexistent at first. That's okay. You can just pretend and still move in a relaxed way, meditating on the feeling of your body. But stay focused on how your body feels during chi gung. Otherwise, you may miss those first faint and subtle sensations of chi.

When you do feel that first glimmer of chi sensation, it may be so faint that it's hard to hang on to it, much less get it to flow. Be patient. Remember, your chi awareness is just waking up. When it does, it is faint and small at first. Compared to your adult dexterity and strength, it's like a toddler. Just like teaching a toddler how to walk, you have to patiently watch and help your chi feeling develop.

In the beginning, your chi gung might be only 5 percent feeling and flow but 95 percent physical motion. It's like holding a toddler's arms up, supporting her weight while she learns how to take her first steps. Over time, your practice may grow to 10 percent feeling and flow with 90 percent physical motion. After several months or years, you may reach a state where your chi has caught up to your muscles, and you can do 50 percent or even 80 percent feeling and flow with progressively less reliance on physical strength and motion. Now that toddler is just holding your little finger, and you can soon let go and watch her walk on her own.

How will you know if you can really feel your chi? Usually, people begin to feel sensations of chi in their fingers, hands, and arms first. Feeling your chi can start out as simply a slightly higher sense of awareness when you put your mind on your arm or your hands. It may be like a tingle inside, or a warmth, a heaviness, or a magnetic or fluid-type feeling when you concentrate and focus on the feeling of your arms or hands. There's no right or wrong. The feeling can vary from person to person and from day to day.

At first, it may be too hard to feel anything at all. That's okay. Pretend for a while and do the best you can. Chances are that you will eventually start to feel something. Whatever it is, use your mind to move that feeling and let your body follow.

The type of moving meditation system taught in authentic chi gung, t'ai chi, and Tao gung is called an *internal* system. That's because we are concerned with what is going on inside our body, our energy, and our feeling when we practice. Conversely, an *external* system of moving focuses only on the physical motion of your body. It stresses strength, repetition, mechanical technique, flexibility, or agility.

If you are doing t'ai chi or chi gung just for exercise, you are using it as an external system. Making this mistake means you'll miss the best part. If you need exercise, you can swim, play tennis, or jog and probably get just as much benefit as t'ai chi or chi gung done only on the physical level. If you use it as an internal system, however, you move your body and your energy. That's how to really get the benefits chi gung can offer. After all, you are not practicing to exercise your body, you are practicing to exercise your energy.

That's why, when studied for self-defense, t'ai chi is called an internal martial art. It is very different than studying karate, tae kwon do, or any of the many other external martial art systems. In an external system, you learn how to use your physical strength, size, agility, and speed to your advantage in managing an opponent. In an internal martial art, like t'ai chi, you learn how to feel, strengthen, flow, and use your energy to manage your opponent. It has nothing to do with the strength, size, and speed of your physical body.

When a t'ai chi master throws, kicks, or punches somebody, he relies very little on strength, speed, or agility. Instead, his internal energy comes out and gives an explosive, extra force to propel his opponent. That chi explosion is what gives the t'ai chi master an edge and why the martial arts application of t'ai chi is called *t'ai chi chuan,* or "grand ultimate fist." It's considered the ultimate martial art, because if you can tap into and use that chi energy, it won't matter if your opponent is physically stronger, bigger, or faster than you. You'll still be able to manage him, because your energy signal is stronger than his, and you can use that energy to provide the force you need to deal with whatever attack he sends your way.

It goes back to the hierarchy of energy levels we discussed before. The energy or chi level can always override or dominate what is happening on the physical level. That's why a chi master using energy can override anything his opponent can do with simple physical-level techniques.

To develop that type of skill in t'ai chi takes many years of strengthening your ability to feel and flow life energy internally. Once you can do that, you can learn to flow it outside your body for chi applications such as martial arts.

You don't have to be interested in martial arts to benefit from learning to flow and move your energy. What if you're a healer, not a fighter? You need to have the same skill that a t'ai chi martial artist has in being able to move your energy and use chi for healing. That includes healing others as well as yourself.

THE POWER OF FEELING AND FLOW IN SELF-HEALING

After we learn to feel and flow our chi, we want to learn how to move the sensation of chi. This is important for self-healing, because we can learn to flow our chi inside our body to where it hurts or where attention is needed.

When you move through your typical day, you rarely feel your body. Can you feel your fourth toe right now? Probably not. But if someone stepped on that toe, then you'd know it was there. You walk and use your feet all day long. You don't even realize it. You are continually unaware of them with no apology. But when your feet hurt, you finally say, "Oh, I'd better take better care of my feet." Unfortunately, that's the only time your feeling and awareness wake up.

Most of the time, I don't feel my feet or toes, stomach, heart, shoulder, my pelvis, knees, or pancreas. Most of us have completely disconnected from our own bodies. We don't feel anymore. We pay a high price for this lack of feeling. Those parts that we cannot or do not feel are like dead zones in our body. If we cannot move our power of feeling and consciousness to them, they may as well be dead to us.

In our practice, we want to learn how to feel our entire body again. We start by feeling those parts we are moving and gradually expand to feel more and more of our body at the same time. For example, in our first few weeks of practicing chi gung, we may be focused on our hands, what they are doing, and where they are going. That's why it's easy to start with trying to actually *feel* our hands.

But we shouldn't stop there. Instead of just feeling our hands, next time we practice, we want to feel the entire sensation of every part of our arm as we move. A few weeks later, we not only hold on to that feeling of our arms, we start to expand our feeling awareness to include the sensation of our shoulders, back, and torso at the same time. Pretty soon, we feel our entire body all at once, even our internal organs. We work toward a global sensation of feeling awareness throughout our physical body.

I often challenge my students, "When you turn to the right, can you turn your liver along with you? When you turn, do you feel the back of your ear turning too?"

If we can't feel a certain area of our body, then we cannot flow our chi there. Many people dream of achieving a level where they can send energy out of their body to another person in healing or martial arts applications. But if you cannot feel your own kidneys or flow energy to them, how can you feel and send energy to someone else who has kidney problems? If you cannot feel and sense what is going on in your own body, how can you feel those subtle signals from your martial arts opponent and sense what he will do in advance so you can dodge his blows or send your energy out to counter him?

If you don't plan on using chi gung for healing others or learning martial arts, why should you want to learn how to feel your entire body? Because you eventually want to be able to flow energy to any point inside yourself. When your clear and calm absolute mind can flow that energy fused with pure feeling, this can initiate or hasten repair and healing to wherever you need it. This is because chi will flow to where your mind and feeling flow.

Using chi for self-healing is simple if you know how to flow with feeling and a pure, calm mind. If you can flow your energy to your knee, you do not have to understand your knee problem mentally, read osteopathic books, think about how to fix it, say affirmations, or visualize anything. You don't need to be a medical expert, because your chi already is. Just sending that healing energy with pure intent and feeling to your knee will be enough for your chi to pick up the information it needs to rally the body's ability to heal itself. Your chi knows what to do.

Even if you do not have any health issues, you should still practice flowing your chi to every part of your body on a regular basis. This allows your chi to patrol around, finding and resolving potential imbalances before they start.

INVEST IN WHAT IS REAL

Do I do moving meditation to pack my brain with new facts or learn something more about chi gung? No. Do I do moving meditation to exercise my muscles? No. I do chi gung moving meditation to remind my life energy of the right way to flow, to remind my system of the "true me."

My thinking is not me. That's outside stuff. Trust me, just like you, I'm an educated intellectual. I know many things. Don't test me. I can talk nonsense with you all day. But even though I know many things, that's not the real me. The sum total of what you think you know is not the real you either, no matter how smart you are.

You have lots of unreal things that you think are part of you. You have your knowledge and education; you have a name that somebody slapped on you at birth; you have a Social Security number; and you probably have a driver's license. Are these things you? No. They have nothing to do with the real you.

If you get sick, can you go change your driver's license number to get better? Can you earn a degree to get better? These have nothing to do with the real you, your life energy. You can only feel and experience the true you by blocking out all that other nonsense.

Let's try another example. When you pinch yourself, it hurts. "Ow! Now that's the real me." That's why feeling and thinking are different. You can use your thoughts and imagination when you begin practicing moving meditation, but eventually you want to go back to real feeling. Feeling can connect to a part of you that is truly real in a way that thinking simply can't.

You want to make sure you are focused on the feeling inside and work with a calm, meditative mind to feel, move, and flow your life energy during chi gung. You can learn a thousand new chi gung forms from a dozen different masters, but if you don't have that feeling of life energy and know how to flow it, you are merely doing slow-motion exercise. That's why it does no good just to copy somebody else's chi gung forms like a monkey-see, monkey-do physical exercise or think that fancier forms will deliver better results.

My students sometimes bring me one or two of the many books written about chi gung or t'ai chi or Tao gung. I tell them that, to really do this, you must get rid of books. You can read forever, but then you end up as one of the victims of education. You can read about swimming all your life and consider yourself an expert on swimming. You can even hold and cherish a deep love for swimming, worshipping it all your life. But if you never get in the water, how can you be a master of swimming?

You must put down your books at some point and practice moving meditation for real. You have to flow. You have to exercise your energy. *You have to do it.*

The old wisdom from the *T'ai Chi Classics* says, "It's right next to you." The truth is within you. You just have to exercise it. If you continue looking for more remote truth, you risk losing everything.

In doing moving meditation or t'ai chi, the real object of your discipline and study is always *you.* I always tell my students, "Chi gung is not your goal. It's just a vehicle." Making that chi connection inside you is your goal, so you can pick up your original life energy signal again. Chi gung and t'ai chi are simply the ways and means that get you to that goal.

7

CLEANING AND RESTORING
YOUR ENERGY: CHI GUNG EXERCISES

THESE EXERCISES ARE like a gift to you. Each time you do them, you benefit. When you don't incorporate this realization into your life, it's as if you give this gift back to me and lose out. Five minutes—or even two— of just one of these chi gung movements gets your chi started back on the right track of moving to help heal internal imbalances.

But remember, just as it hurts to forget, disregard, and *not* do this practice, it can hurt your life energy to do *too much*. If you approach chi gung with a strong, ambitious, willful determination to practice five, seven, or even twelve hours a day, it can backfire on you. The book *T'ai Chi Classics* says, "Not too much, not too little." We have to stay gentle and relaxed. Working to the point of tension or pain, trying too hard, or coveting progress too much can all block and damage your chi. It's like cooking food. If you undercook it, that's no good. But cooking until it burns and is no longer edible is just as bad. Too much equals not enough; both equal no good.

This is a training program. It is conditioning. It is reprogramming. What does reprogramming mean? It means your current program isn't working right, so you put in a new program. But you can't completely get rid of your body's old program, so what do you do?

A bad program is like poison in your system. To get rid of it, you must dilute it. If I cannot extract poison out of a bucket of water, what do I do? I keep adding more water to thin it out. Likewise, if I keep adding more and more good programming to my system, it can dilute the bad programming. It's a little like how chi gung will work.

You do this moving meditation a little bit here, a little bit there. It's not a magic pill that works all at once, but a reprogramming process that accumulates over time. For that reason, it's best to treat chi gung as a lifestyle. You can practice every morning or during any spare time, like when you're standing in line at the airport or sitting in the car. If I'm waiting in line at the post office, I can take one or two minutes, whatever spare time I have, to feel my lower stomach and flow my energy just a little.

In respect to reaching the goal of restoring life energy, the *quality* of your practice is far more important than the *quantity*. You can practice the right way for three seconds and get much further than if you practice the wrong way for three years. Everything I've mentioned about using feeling combined with a pure, calm mind contributes to a high quality of practice.

Some people wonder why we do moving meditation so slowly. It's because we are so busy. When you do chi gung the right way, you have to concentrate so you can feel and not lose track of your life energy. You become busy feeling and flowing that energy so you can get the most out of it.

Do you know how they tortured prisoners in the old days? They would make them eat their food very fast. That way, the prisoners could not taste or enjoy their food. It was more like force-feeding. Everyone knows that if you chew food for a long time, it has more flavor and gives you more nourishment and enjoyment.

Following the same idea, if I do chi gung quickly, I will miss the chance to savor the feeling and get all the benefit out of it. If I do chi gung or t'ai chi slowly, I can feel everything going on and get the most out of it. If I move very slowly and carefully, deeply aware of what I'm doing, I get to chew on that feeling. That's how to harvest the best essence of chi gung, t'ai chi, or Tao gung.

Since the goal is to rejoin your mind and life energy, it's important to bring a clean, calm mind to all of these exercises. Do your best to quiet your mind and put away any distractions or concerns. If you are upset, angry, and agitated, it is better to do something else first, like walking around the block, working on something physical, or resolving whatever problem is aggravating you. You'll get more benefit if you are able to calm your mind down before trying these moving meditation exercises.

Why do I keep repeating "pure, clean, and calm mind?" Remember, we are trying to duplicate the state of our single cell or embryo in order to wake up that original energy. Is an embryo anxious, angry, agitated, or distracted? No, it just feels and flows calmly through each moment of its being. This is the original state of the mind—simple, clean, direct, and calm. By imitating the mental condition of a baby or an embryo, over a long period of practice, we actually start to feel like a baby feels.

The exercises that follow are a mixture of chi gung and Tao gung moving meditation forms. They are designed to open up the internal chi flow within your body and embed your chi with new programming that will bring it back to a condition of greater harmony. At first, don't worry about getting every form or movement precisely. It's more important just to *do* it as best you can rather than to do it perfectly.

Over time and with practice, your body will acclimate and feel how to do the moves correctly. Re-read the instructions for the form from time to time to correct yourself. If there are any instructions you don't understand, forget about them and just imitate the pictures as closely as possible. These exercises are not designed to bring more stress into your life by making you worry about too many details; they are meant to get you started with a program of simple moving meditation exercises. If you have a sincere attitude, you will soon get on the right track, even if you feel clumsy at first.

Tan Tien Meditation

Here is a simple but powerful meditation that you can do almost any-where and anytime. You can even adapt this standing meditation and do it while sitting, reclining, or walking. You can also do it while waiting in line, standing around at the office, or anytime you want to bring your-self back to a more centered feeling of harmony.

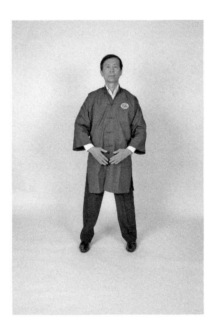

First locate the center of each palm. Don't just think about it or look at it; really feel the center point. Here's a trick you can use to help. Lightly touch the center of your palm with the opposite index finger, then pull your finger away and see if you can still hang on to feeling that point. Do the same with the other palm.

Once you can feel the center of each palm, bring your hands in front of your lower stomach area, right below your navel (a), and beam the center of each palm inward toward one point inside your lower stomach. Aim for just below your navel and a few inches inside. Although your palms are close to and facing your lower stomach, they do not touch each other, and they do not touch your stomach. You can keep your eyes open if you wish. However, closing your eyes will help you concentrate on that point inside your lower stomach.

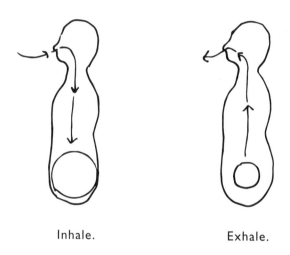

Inhale.   Exhale.

As you breathe, inhale and exhale from that spot in your lower stomach. Try to feel as if there is a ball in that spot. As you inhale, that imaginary ball expands very slightly (b). As you exhale, it gets smaller again (c).

As you inhale, move your hands slightly out and away from your stomach, following and expanding with the ball. As you exhale, again follow the shrinking ball and bring your hands back closer to your stomach. But remember, whether you're inhaling or exhaling, expanding or contracting the ball, your hands never actually touch your stomach. They always stay a few inches away.

Really concentrate on the center of your palms beaming toward the center of your lower stomach—your tan tien. Feel how the imaginary ball in your lower stomach area expands and contracts as you inhale and exhale.

Do this meditation for as long and as often as you like. When you are finished, gradually open your eyes. Spread your fingers, and think about your elbows. Let your elbows pull your hands away from your stomach so they can fall gently down at your sides.

The Benefits of Tan Tien Meditation

This seems like such a simple meditation and it is, but it is also one of the most important. Why? Improving our ability to connect with our tan tien is a huge part of our journey to restore our life energy. This exercise helps in the following ways:

- To train our energy to go back to its origin, that place in the lower stomach just behind the navel where life began

- To learn how to work with an imaginary ball of energy originating inside the lower stomach

- To pay attention to and coordinate our motion with our breathing

Each of these are fundamental building blocks for almost all chi gung, t'ai chi, and Tao gung forms.

The tan tien is where the center of original life energy began. It's the place we need to go to wake up that original programming we are looking for. It isn't an anatomical spot, meaning you won't find it if you cut open someone's abdomen. It is, however, an energy center that houses the original memory of the Te inside us.

You may actually sense something in your lower stomach area as you do this exercise. That sensation may move, grow, and change over time. Remember, your tan tien is not a physical, stationary location; rather, it is a living, moving field of energy.

Lining up our hands in front of our stomach and beaming the center of our palms inward is a trick we use to guide the mind more easily to the tan tien. Our mind is very connected to our hands. As we grow up, our mental acuity and focus quickly migrates to our hands so we can use them with seamless coordination. Humans are known for great dexterity—typing, writing, fixing things. The mind develops a sharp, firm connection to each hand. Our hands are like the utmost extensions, or antennae, of our mind. Therefore, it is easy to use our mind to flow our concentration and chi to our hands.

By working with both hands in this exercise, we are also bringing together both the right and left hemispheres of our brain and teaching them to focus together on one spot. That spot is where they were once joined together, existing as one before they split in two. Tan tien meditation works to bring those two hemispheres of the brain into greater communication, cooperation, and harmony with each other.

When we connect our mind to our hands by focusing on the center of each palm and then bring the palms in to focus on our tan tien, it creates a type of shortcut to bring our mental energy back to the center of our life energy. We use those antennae to beam all our mind energy inward. By bringing our hands and the unified concentration of our whole mind, back to our center, we are training our mind and energy to return home. We want to reprogram them to go to the place where our life energy originated. Remember, in chi gung, we want to re-create a younger signal—powerful, loud, and clear. That's why we keep going back to the tan tien where that spark of life first came into this world.

You can speed up the process of restoring your life energy if you make an effort to revert to this form any time you find yourself sitting or standing around. If you are in the grocery line, waiting for a bus, or sitting in your office chair, feel the center of each palm and bring them in front of your tan tien. Concentrate on the feeling of expanding and contracting your imaginary ball inward and outward with each inhalation and exhalation. You can be discreet and keep your movements very small, so no one will detect that you are actually doing moving meditation. Simple but powerful! In fact, this meditation form is so important and so effective, that every single chi gung, t'ai chi, and Tao gung exercise begins and ends with it.

We'll explore more about the importance of the tan tien in the next meditation form.

Advanced Tan Tien Meditation

If you have some quiet time and would like to go deeper into meditation to restore your life energy, try this advanced version of a tan tien meditation. This advanced version is especially important for people seeking to use chi gung for spiritual development. It's also great for those who want a new and uniquely rewarding and revitalizing method of meditation.

Start with the same meditation exercise described in the previous section, locating the center of each palm and bringing them together in front of your lower stomach to beam toward your tan tien. Relax as you inhale and exhale, expanding and contracting that imaginary ball inside your stomach. Remember, although you are standing in one place and focusing on one spot, this is still moving meditation. You are moving inward and outward, following your breathing and the ball as it expands and contracts.

Right now the ball in your lower stomach may still be imaginary, but at some point, it will not be. If you are very relaxed, you soon may actually feel and sense a real ball of energy. Don't worry, that is a mark of progress—chi awareness. Stay relaxed and gently work to cooperate with and follow that real sensation as it expands and contracts.

While you are in your meditation, beaming the center of your palms inward, close your eyes and visualize that you are using your power of sight to look inside and down into your body toward the same spot. Concentrating on that one point, ask yourself, "Can I see anything there?" This will help focus your intention on that spot.

Next, pay attention to your ears. Use that listening power, pull it inside, and beam it down toward your center. Can you hear anything inside?

Now pay attention to your nose. Aim your ability to smell down toward the same spot. Focus all the power of your nose, all of its attention, on your lower stomach. Can you smell anything?

Next, pretend the back or root of your tongue actually starts all the way down inside your lower stomach. Use your power of taste from that imaginary root, to see if your tongue can taste anything in your tan tien.

Now pull in your sense of feeling from your skin. Pretend that this sense from all over your body is now aimed inward toward your center. Can you feel anything?

If you find your mind starting to wander during this process, don't worry. Gently remind it to come back. Give it permission to think but to think only about that one spot! While you are focused on that spot, swallow gently. Feel that swallow as it moves down to the same spot. This will help you focus even more.

See how many of these different senses you can pull in at once to concentrate on that same tan tien point. If you lose concentration on one (or more) of your senses, gently pull it back. Stay in this meditation for as long as you like and are comfortable.

When you are finished, gradually open your eyes. Spread your fingers, and think about your elbows. Let your elbows pull your hands away from your stomach so they can fall gently down at your sides.

Benefits of Advanced Tan Tien Meditation

This is a very powerful meditation because we are bringing each of our sensory powers back to their origin, the center of life energy. After all, where did the eye and the power of sight originally come from? Our first single cell. Where did the ear originally come from? Our first single cell. All of our senses' root potential started in that cell and reside in that original center of life energy. By bringing them all back to their origin, we are once again programming ourselves to go home.

The original energy in our tan tien, that power of the first single cell, is far more potent than any of our senses. After all, an eye cell such as a specialized rod or cone cell that can perceive light or color, or a taste bud on the tongue, are no longer stem cells. They gave up that stem cell power precisely so they could perform a single function. Our sensory cells and sensory function have stepped down from that power of original life energy. We want to bring them back to it.

As you go through this exercise, remember that you can't actually see, hear, or taste your original energy. Such energy has no smell, no color, no sound. Lao Tzu said in the *Tao Te Ching,* "Look, but you cannot see it—it is formless. Listen, but you cannot hear it—it transcends sound."[1]

However, during this meditation, you may have sensory experiences. You may see color or light. You may hear something or smell different aromas. You may have any of several different experiences that seem marvelous. This is all normal. But when my students report such occurrences, I tell them, "Don't interpret. Keep going." Why? Because if you can see, smell, or taste something, it's still not that original energy you are looking for. The core of original energy comes from the Tao. Lao Tzu describes the Tao as *bu xiao,* which means "nothing like it." So if, in your meditation, you experience something you are able to interpret and describe, gently keep meditating to penetrate even deeper into your tan tien. This means that while you look, listen, smell, taste, and feel, no matter what you find, you keep going, always looking for something purer and deeper.

If your desire in meditation is to look for something or achieve something, you're in trouble. You stop your progress right there. Meditation is meant to help you give up, to purify, to reduce. You may even think to yourself, "I want to see God," or "I want to see Light," or "I want to learn something." Even such noble desires can block your real achievement, because by holding such desires, you set a limit for yourself. One meaning of *t'ai chi* is "no limit." When there's a limit, then you aren't able to experience the unlimited nature of the Tao. You have to keep working to approach your meditation with absolute mind, using your pure feeling and pure awareness, with no expectations.

It is okay to experience color, tone, or different flavors, but do not forget to go back to the root, meaning your Te. That's why the *Tao Te Ching* says, "The five colors blind your eye. The five sounds deafen your ear. The five flavors ruin your taste. Too much hunting and games confuse your mind."[2] It's your core energy that enables you to hear, see, and sense everything. But don't be confused. You don't want to be distracted by the flowers of that core energy; you want to keep going to the source.

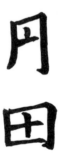

Chinese character for *tan tien.*

These two Chinese characters comprise the term *tan tien.* In ancient Chinese, *tan* means the sun and moon, or yin and yang, joined together; *tien* means a fertile field, like a farmer's field. The message hidden within the original Chinese characters is thus "planting the sun and moon together in a fertile field." Here's a short history of how these two characters evolved in the Chinese language and how we can extract important meaning from them for our meditation.

In the earliest history of the Chinese language, pictograms were carved on bone to record important events and stories. Eventually, characters evolved that were carved into wood or bamboo; later still, they were printed on silk. After the invention of paper, more and more

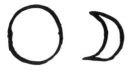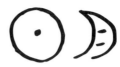

Earliest carvings on bone evolving into a pictograph.

The present day character for *ming* (brightness),
looking less like a sun and moon.

Ming: sun and moon.

Ming: sun and moon,
superimposed.

Early form of *tan*.

Present-day *tan*.

characters evolved, and more and more cultural records were written down.

The evolution of the character for *tan* started with the evolution of the word for "brightness," or *ming*. On bone, it would have been carved with a plain sun and moon together. Gradually, a word began to form, and the pictograph changed over time.

The sun and moon were the brightest objects ancient people knew, so putting them together in this way meant brightness. How did these two symbols meaning brightness evolve into the character for *tan*?

Tan means the joining of the sun and moon together, the joining of yin and yang, or the ultimate brightness. Watch what happens when you gradually start to superimpose the symbol for the sun over the symbol for the moon in the ming pictograph. It evolves into the current character we know as *tan*.

This is the secret meaning of the word *tan*. It means sun and moon together, or an ultimate brightness that is much higher than ming. Where is this ultimate brightness located? Let's look at the character for *tien*, or "fertile field." You can easily see this familiar representation if you imagine flying over a rural landscape and looking down at a section of farmland.

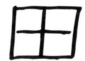

Tien character.

Your lower stomach area is where Taoists believe that the universal life energy enters the body. It is the center of fertility where a woman's body can nurture new life. It is also the place in our bodies from which our own life energy unfolds from our embryonic being until today.

So the deep meaning within the compound character for *tan tien* is that your left and right hands are yin and yang, the sun and moon. Your mental and sensory perceptions are bright and shining and full of energy like the sun and moon. The fertile field is your lower stomach. You want to plant the sun and moon in the fertile field by beaming your right and left hand inward, along with all your senses, to the center of your lower stomach.

RESTORING YOUR LIFE ENERGY

In another analogy, your senses are like the flowers of that original seed of life energy. You want to bring all those senses together again and concentrate them, like pulling in all those flowers and planting them like one concentrated seed in the "fertile field" of your lower stomach. Focusing all your attention, senses, and hands into that one point inside is like planting a seed. This is the meditation that the Chinese character for *tan tien* describes.

Where we put our concentration matters in our life. Putting it on our tan tien, on our life energy, can reap great benefits. Constantly putting our concentration outside ourselves, on things that are not worthwhile and that pollute our life energy, can hurt us. That's why the character for *tan tien* advises us to put our seed of concentration in the fertile field of our life energy.

This advice is strikingly similar to the parable of the sower in the New Testament, in which Jesus advised his followers to sow their seed in fertile soil to reap true rewards. He warned them that seed sown on rocky ground would never take root and would wither away. If their seed fell among thorns, the thorns would choke any growth. If the seed were scattered by the wayside, birds would steal it.

Look at your life and all the things that compete for your concentration and attention—television programs, video games, worries, fears, news headlines, and so on. How similar are your life's distractions to thorns or rocky soil? How many things are like birds that steal your focus, attention, and time, preventing you from meditating and making that connection with your life energy? What do you reap by focusing your attention on these outside things? Why not plant your seed in fertile soil instead?

When you take even a few minutes away from distractions that steal your "seed" and instead put them into a few minutes of chi gung meditation, it's like planting that seed in fertile soil. If you make this practice a regular part of your lifestyle, your seed can take root, allowing your chi connection to bear fruit, healing and restoring your body, mind, and spirit.

How can such a simple practice, done for a few minutes every day, help so much? Consider another analogy in the stories Jesus told. He said if you have faith like a mustard seed, you can move mountains! What is faith but pure, sincere, and focused concentration on the ultimate truth of that One Universal Energy, Tao, or God? This is the type of spirit and attitude you can bring to your tan tien meditation. Say to yourself, "I let go of all the cares and distractions of life. I just want to concentrate, connect, and feel that pure life energy inside. I want to bring everything I am into that tiny center spot so I can be one with that piece of God inside me."

When all of your concentrated senses and mind join together and focus on one small point, it most approximates the original condition of your single cell. Because you have re-created a condition close to original life energy by improving your ability to do tan tien meditation, you have a much better chance of reconnecting with that energy.

At the chi gung level, this exercise helps us regain a deep sense of centeredness, as we pull all those disconnected pieces of ourselves back together. It sends that strong signal of centeredness and harmony back to our chi, so it can circulate the message throughout our entire body. At a more advanced level, this exercise is part of the practice and work that serious Tao gung practitioners use to drill down to their Te, that piece of original energy inside.

Circulating Feeling Awareness throughout the Body

Here's another meditation exercise you can do whenever you have some spare quiet time. You can even do it as you lie down at bedtime.

While you are standing, seated, or lying down, calm your mind and focus on the feeling in your tan tien. Concentrate until you can really feel that area.

Now, in a smooth and continuous manner, move that feeling and concentration to the side and slowly down one leg. Make a smooth and continuous path; don't jump from one spot to the next. Pretend you are tracing a line or following a pathway with your feeling.

Move the feeling from your thigh slowly down to your knee, your calf, your ankle, your foot, and into each toe. Stop and spend some time feeling each body part. Move the energy up to your tan tien again, slowly and smoothly in a continuous path. Now move that feeling awareness over to the other side and down the opposite leg to your knee, foot, and toes, then back to your tan tien.

Now move the feeling inside and around your torso, searching for each internal organ and stopping to feel and concentrate on each one. Maintain a calm attitude, perhaps even send a feeling message: "I'm sorry I've ignored you for so long." Use your feeling to let each part of your body know how much you value and appreciate it, thanking it for all it does. No need to talk or use language, just hold that intention inside your sincere feeling as you move your energy around inside your body.

After you have explored the inside of your torso, return the feeling to your tan tien. Now move it down to your tailbone and come up through your spine. Slowly try to feel each vertebra. As you come up to your shoulder area, send that feeling out and down the inside of one of your arms, through your elbow, down to your wrist, hand, and fingers. Smoothly return to your shoulder area, and cross over to the other shoulder, moving your concentrated feeling down the opposite arm.

When you are finished with both arms, send your feeling energy up through your spine and the back of your neck, over the top of your head, and down your face, your eyes and ears and jaw. Continue moving the feeling down the front of your neck, stopping to feel inside your throat, larynx, and esophagus. Continue to move your energy down the front of your chest and stomach and back to your tan tien.

This process can take a long time. Don't worry about too many details at first. You do not have to perform a complete, anatomically accurate tour of your body. Down the road, you can add more time and detail while you do this exercise. If you only have a little time, you can start at your tan tien and only flow the energy through your torso. Or perhaps you'd like to flow only to each arm, spending a little extra time at the elbows. You can adapt this exercise so that you flow your feeling awareness to any place you wish.

Benefits of Circulating Feeling Awareness throughout the Body

Even though you may be just standing, sitting, or lying there, if you are moving that feeling and concentration you are still practicing moving meditation. How? Wherever your feeling awareness and mind go, your chi tends to follow. So by moving your concentrated feeling awareness, you are learning how to move your energy.

This exercise is excellent for slowly developing the ability to feel your chi. The simple act of moving in a continuous pathway up and down each limb, up the spine, or down and through each finger opens up energy channels in your body that may be blocked or to which you've grown insensitive.

The important thing to remember is to maintain a slow, continuous, and unbroken path while moving your feeling. You cannot just jump from your lower abdomen and put your attention on your sore foot. No, to send life energy there, you must first start at your tan tien, feel that life energy, and send it down to your foot in a continuous line of flow. Remember, life energy does not jump or jerk; it flows. That's how your body was formed—by flow, gradually building itself section by section. So to heal, you have to flow your energy from your tan tien through each part along that same pathway, section to section.

This exercise also helps fuse that damaging separation between your mind, body, and chi. Most of us have spent so much time focusing our attention outside that we've lost touch with our internal feeling and the chi connection inside that keeps our organs and bodily systems working together in harmony. We are like strangers to our own body. Now is your chance to get reacquainted and turn that focus inward; apologize to your body; and bring your physical body back in touch with your mind, feeling, and chi.

Additionally, when you perform this special meditation, it's as if you are "on patrol." The patrolling of that concentrated feeling and life energy can help chase out any bad stuff or alert your system to internal areas that need attention. Even if you are not consciously aware of it, your energy will pick up what it needs to know to start rebalancing.

Again, as you circulate your energy, if you pick up any information, see anything, hear anything, feel anything unusual, do not interpret it. Do not stop and fight with anything or draw conclusions based on your experience. Keep calm and keep flowing. Let go and let your original energy do its job.

Flowing Your Energy through Your Feet

Here's a simple exercise you can do whenever you find yourself standing around. You can do it in a manner so that nobody else will notice that you are actually practicing chi gung moving meditation. In addition to flowing your internal energy, you'll find that doing this exercise will help you stand for longer periods of time without tiring.

This is a standing exercise in which you will place your concentration on the soles of your feet. While you are standing in one place, with your feet parallel and comfortably apart, focus your concentration and feeling on a point on the bottom of your left big toe. Even though both feet are firmly on the ground, feel as though your weight is shifting inside to land firmly on this point.

Now move this attention slowly and seamlessly to the left, flowing it to a point under the second left toe (a). Now flow your feeling and concentration along a continuous line to a point under the third toe, the fourth, and finally the little toe, until you've shifted your attention through each (b). As you flow your concentration and feeling from point to point under each toe, sense your weight shifting along this path as well.

Now flow your attention along the outside of your left sole in a continuous path, until you reach a point under your left heel (c).

Now flow your attention around the heel to the inside of your foot and outward through a point on the floor right in the middle of your feet (d). Next, move it up to a point on the bottom of your right big toe (e).

Repeat the same series of flow motions from point to point under your right foot. Start by flowing from a point under the right big toe to a point under the second toe, then the third, fourth, and little toes (f). Flow along the outside edge of your right sole to a point underneath your right heel (g).

Flow around the heel, up to the center point on the floor between your feet, and back up to the point on the bottom of your left toe, where you began (h). Notice as you flow your feeling along this path that you are tracing an infinity symbol. That may help you remember the path of flow in this exercise.

You can also reverse the flow and start with a point under your right toe and flow clockwise in the same manner. Repeat in a smooth, continuous figure eight for as long as you like, alternating the flow from clockwise to counterclockwise.

At first, it may help to shift your weight very slightly and slowly as you follow this path, but as time goes on, you will no longer want this shift to be physical. You do *not* want to end up rocking your body around and around. Ideally, you want to flow your energy and shift your weight in such a manner that anyone looking at you wouldn't be able to detect what you're doing. The shift is primarily internal. You want the sensation that you are shifting the energy inside your body as you follow the figure eight pattern. It can help to imagine your body as a bottle full of heavy liquid, and you are slowly swirling that liquid inside you, feeling it flow in harmony with the path you are imagining at the soles of your feet.

Be careful not to lose your balance when you practice this. For the first few times, it may help to hold on to a railing or the back of a chair for support. If you feel off balance, follow the points on your feet with your imagination only; don't try to shift anything at all. You can also place your feet farther apart if this is more comfortable and helps you keep your balance. This will not diminish the benefits of the exercise.

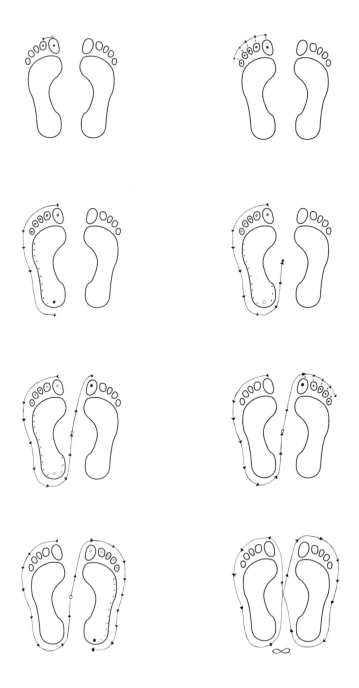

RESTORING YOUR LIFE ENERGY

Benefits of Flowing Energy through Your Feet

Once again, it is important to remember not to jump from point to point; you want to flow seamlessly. Lao Tzu says that the Tao is like water. You don't see water in a river jump from here to there; it flows. Flow your feeling from one point to another. Make your attention, your feeling, and your energy like a river, flowing from one toe to the next, around a series of imaginary points in an infinite loop.

In addition to the benefit of calming meditation, this exercise can help you increase your physical balance. Is that because you are strengthening your muscles? No, it is because you are restoring your sensitivity and awareness in the soles of your feet.

Most of us walk around all day, relying on our feet and abusing them terribly without a second thought. The only time we feel and consider our feet is when they hurt. Yet through this exercise, we can wake up the connection and the feeling in our feet. This ability is important as we get older, since it helps us sense when we are off balance, thus preventing falls. (Research studies have shown that t'ai chi improves foot sensitivity in diabetics and can help prevent falls in older adults.)

Additionally, the feet are what acupuncturists and Oriental medicine practitioners refer to as a microcosm of the entire body. Different points or areas of the feet can be needled or massaged to bring stimulation and healing to every part of the body. These are called *reflexology points*. Perhaps you have heard of or received a reflexology massage.

Because you are flowing your energy through so many points on your feet with this exercise, it is like you are giving yourself an energy massage. You are stimulating and bringing restorative energy to many different systems in your body just by concentrating on your feet.

In this exercise, you may be barely able to feel the surface of the soles of your feet at first. That's okay; do the best you can. Over time, you may be able to zero in on the front of your sole and not the whole surface. This is progress! Soon you may be able to detect and isolate your feeling to a surface as big as a nickel under your big toe, then a dime, then the head of a pin. There is no limit to how small you can go. The smaller the point, the better your ability to focus your feeling and awareness with a pure mind.

With all of our moving meditation exercises, whether we are using the center of our palms, the tan tien spot in our lower stomach, or points on our feet, we try to improve our concentration until we can focus on one point. We do this for a reason, even though it is hard. When we focus on a broad area or large surface, our energy is diffused. It's like a lightbulb shining in all directions. Yes, there is energy, but it is widely dispersed. However, if we can focus that light through one single point, it becomes a laser beam, which is much more powerful and can penetrate deeply. It can carry and deliver that healing signal we're looking for. The smaller we can make this point, the more energy our sincerity and concentration will deliver to it.

Don't worry about matching up your imaginary points in this exercise to actual acupuncture points on a chart somewhere. Just meditate, flow, and enjoy. Trust that the chi flow through your feet will gradually open up the flow inside your entire body.

Remember, you aren't only flowing energy through all those points on your feet. Because you are also trying to shift and feel your internal energy as you move around and around, like swirling heavy liquid in a bottle, you are learning to flow energy throughout your whole body. A version of this exercise called Non–Arms Training is used by advanced t'ai chi martial artists. They can sometimes practice for hours, just swirling the sensation of energy in their bodies in any and all directions without lifting or using their legs or arms. It's a powerful method to train their chi to go to any point in their bodies at will.

Clean Your Energy

FORM ONE

Here is the first of two chi gung exercises that you can do to help clean your energy of negative debris that you may pick up in daily life. You might enjoy it when you get home from work, brushing off the stress of the day. But remember, never do any moving meditation when you are angry or upset. Give yourself a chance to calm down first, so you can connect to your life energy with a pure, calm mind. Then your cleaning work will be much more effective.

Every round of moving meditation, every exercise, always starts with your hands in front of your tan tien. The same is true for energy-cleaning chi gung. Stand in the same position as for tan tien meditation; take a few moments as you relax and calm your mind (a). Gently following your breathing in and out can help you settle down inside.

Now imagine that an invisible ball of energy is beginning to grow beneath your palms, expanding outward from your tan tien. As it expands, it pushes your palms outward, so they follow its expanding motion (b).

As the imaginary ball keeps expanding, let your hands float out and up in a big arch to follow the curve of the ball. At first, you cradle the ball just outside your lower stomach, but as it grows, your palms—still pointing toward each other—rise up along the curve until they are as high as your head (c).

Let the expanding ball grow so big that it engulfs you. Keep following the surface of the expanding energy ball with your arms and hands until they are over your head (d). Remember that your arms, hands, and palms should never touch each other or your body; they are always at a slight distance.

Now that you are fully inside your imaginary ball of energy, move your hands up and over the back of your head and down to the nape of your neck (e). Remember, don't touch! Brush down the back of your head, leaving space between your palms and your body so the energy can do its work. Imagine that you are cleaning and clearing out all the energy inside and/or clinging to your body along the path you are tracing with your hands.

Once you've brushed down to the nape of your neck, use the tips of your elbows to slowly pull your fingertips and palms apart (f). Move slowly and with feeling.

Pull your hands just far enough apart so that your fingertips can move forward along and around your neck and come back together (but don't touch) in front of the notch in your collarbone (g).

Slowly brush down the center of your torso with both palms, brushing and beaming energy, full of feeling. Move your hands down the front of your body (h).

When you've brushed down the length of your torso, bring your hands to rest again in front of your tan tien (i). Spend some time here, beaming the center of your palms inward to that point inside your stomach. Gently move your hands in and out as you inhale and exhale, following your expanding and contracting energy. You can repeat this exercise as often as you like.

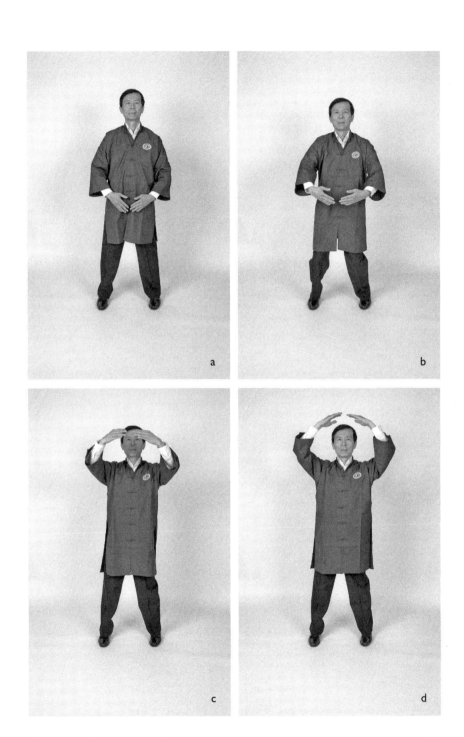

a

b

c

d

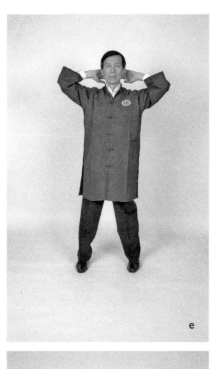

e

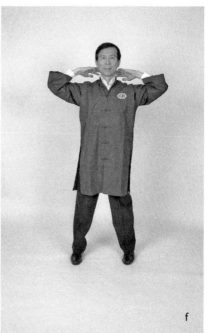

f

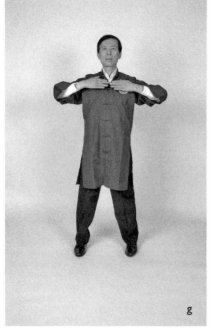

g

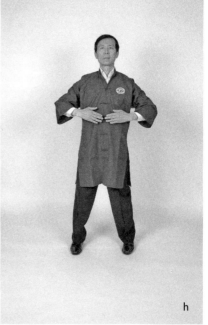

h

RESTORING YOUR LIFE ENERGY

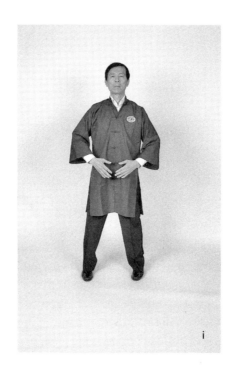

i

Clean Your Energy

FORM TWO

You can also do this second chi gung exercise to help clean your energy. Try to do it on both the right and left sides of your body. If you wish, you can move very slowly and stop awhile at each major joint—such as the shoulder, elbow, and wrist—and gently circle your palm a few times before moving down to the next. This will really help open your energy pathways and bring healing flow to each area.

Once again, you start in a standing position with both palms facing your tan tien (a). This gives you a chance to calm down and focus on that center of life energy in your lower stomach.

Slowly move one palm in back of the other so your hands line up in front of your tan tien (b). Do not let your hands touch each other, and do not let the inside palm touch your stomach. They should be close together but with some space between them. Hold your palms here, gently moving them slightly apart and together again as you inhale and exhale. This charges them up for the next step.

Pretend that the inside palm closest to your stomach is filling up with and holding a small ball of energy that is expanding and splitting itself out from that imaginary ball inside your tan tien. Slowly start to move the second ball upward, and follow along with your palm to help (c). It may feel like you are pushing the ball with your palm at first. Later, you will be able to move it with just your feeling and merely follow along with your palm.

While your palm slowly and continuously moves that imaginary ball of energy up the middle of your torso to your heart, keep your opposite palm facing your tan tien (d). One ball is moving while the one inside your lower stomach stays still. This creates a yin and yang condition that generates a lot of power. Remember, don't allow either palm to touch your body. Keep both at a slight distance to give the energy enough room to work. Just like a spark plug needs a gap in order to generate a spark, touching your body during this exercise is like short-circuiting that power—the energy drops.

Once your palm and the ball of energy reach a point near the center of your upper chest, look toward the shoulder opposite to your raised hand (e). Because life energy will follow where you focus, looking toward your shoulder helps encourage your energy to flow in that direction. At the same time, start to feel the ball moving toward your shoulder while your palm gently pushes or follows it.

As your palm and energy move to the side and brush over your shoulder, feel your shoulder rise ever so slightly, as if to greet that energy (f). You can pause to circle your palm around your shoulder a few times if you like, then gently start to brush the ball of energy down your upper arm. Remember to flow in a smooth, continuous path; don't jump or lose your feeling.

Flow the energy down your upper arm and over your elbow (g). Follow the direction you are flowing with your eyes. As you flow down, your arm starts to gently rise as if it wants to meet the energy. Bring that ball over your elbow. Once again, you can circle your palm over your elbow a few times to help open the energy flow in this important joint. When you are ready, resume your flow by beginning to brush down your forearm.

As you watch your palm brush down your forearm, your forearm rises to meet your energy (h). Keep brushing that ball of energy down until you reach your wrist. If you like, you can pause here to circle your palm a few times around your wrist.

When you are finished flowing through the wrist, flow your energy ball over the top of your opposite hand (i). As you gently flow over each row of knuckle joints, your hand relaxes and curves, rising upward slightly to greet the energy. Remember, your brushing palm never touches your other hand but stays slightly distant. If you like, you can pause and circle your palm a bit over each row of knuckle joints to open the energy flow through your fingers. This takes a lot of relaxation and concentration.

As you brush down your fingers and reach your fingertips, brush all that accumulated energy off, slightly downward and away from yourself, imagining that you are sending it into infinity (j). Let the feeling and the energy ball go. Let go of your cares, worries, and negativity, allowing them to float off and away.

After you've let the energy go, slowly bring both palms out, around, and down (k).

End with your palms back in front of your tan tien (l). Meditate here for a little while.

When you are ready, you can bring the other palm inside, closer to your tan tien, and repeat the same exercise on the opposite side of your body (m–t).

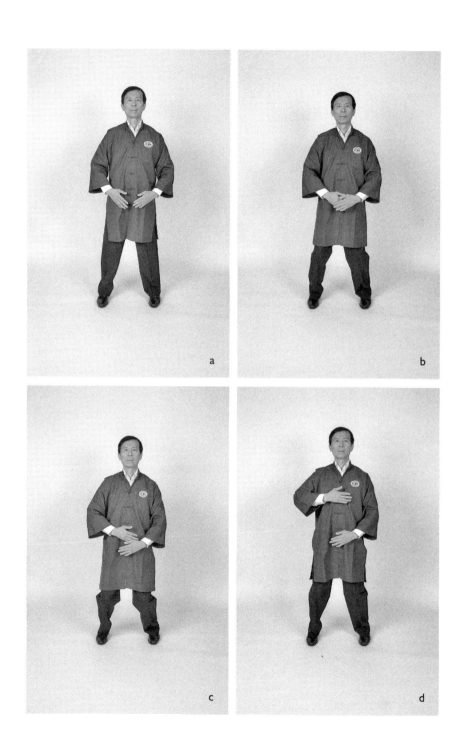

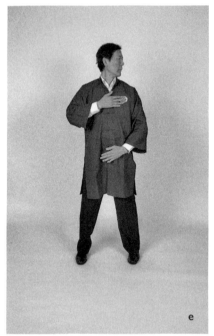

e

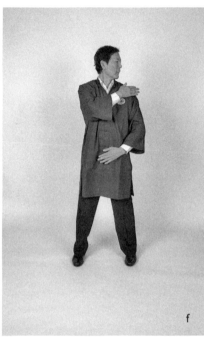

f

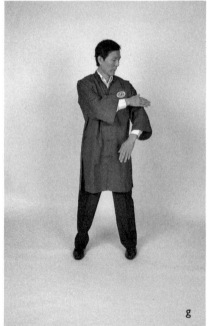

g

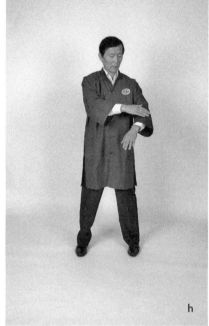

h

RESTORING YOUR LIFE ENERGY

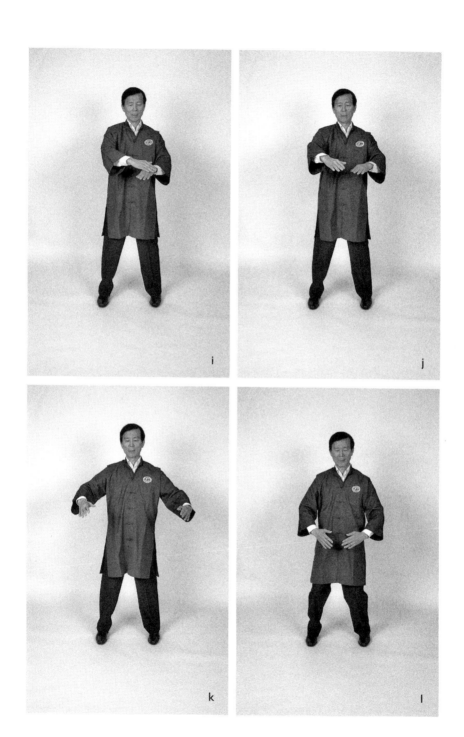

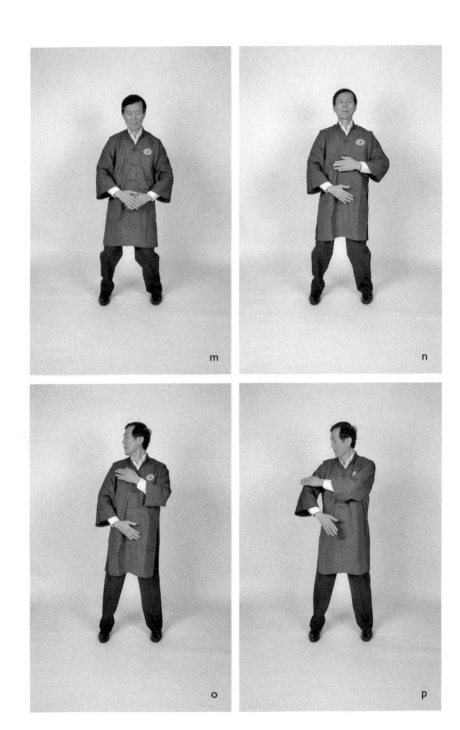

RESTORING YOUR LIFE ENERGY

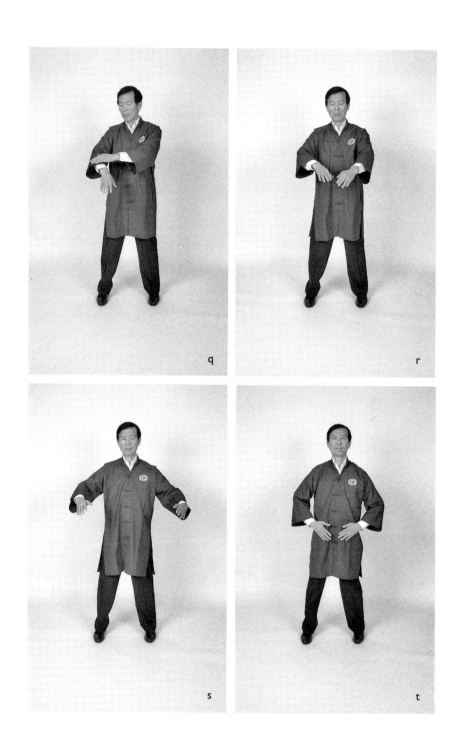

q

r

s

t

Benefits of Cleaning Your Energy: Forms One and Two

When you place your palms in front of your lower stomach and connect their center points to your tan tien, you are charging up the ball of energy inside. Some of that energy remains in your palms as you move away from the tan tien and go through these cleaning forms. You may even feel an energy sensation brushing along the surface of your skin as your palms move up, over, around, and down again, even though your palms aren't touching your body.

In both of these cleaning forms, your palms follow major energy pathways, or meridians, inside your body. By moving slowly and with feeling, you help to open and push energy through these pathways, encouraging your chi to flow.

Your energy must keep flowing to remain clean and vibrant. If a body of water has no flow, it becomes stagnant and cannot support life. Flow keeps the water clean and fresh. Doing these two exercises on a regular basis will help you keep your energy clean, flowing, and refreshed.

Charge-Up Form

In previous exercises, we expanded a ball of energy out from our tan tien in the lower stomach. In Charge-Up Form, we will expand that ball until it is so big that it floats up and expands out to touch the entire universe. It is especially important to practice this form when you feel calm and content and to practice in a peaceful, pleasant environment. Skip this exercise when you are upset, angry, or somewhere that is chaotic or negative.

As always, you begin your moving meditation by calming your mind and focusing on your tan tien, with the center of your palms beaming inward toward that center spot in your lower stomach (a).

From your tan tien, allow a ball of energy to expand outward to fill your palms (b). Move them slowly away from you as you cradle the expanding ball. It's okay if your ball is imaginary to start with, but don't be surprised if someday you really feel something there. That will mean that you've increased your chi awareness.

Imagine the ball of energy expanding even more, requiring both of your arms to hold it; let them rise to accommodate that expansion (c). It may look like you are embracing a big beach ball.

As that ball keeps expanding, it grows lighter like an inflated balloon and rises up as it grows. Raise your arms to keep holding on to the ball, and start to move them apart to accommodate the ball's expansion (d).

Now that imaginary ball is so big, the best you can do is cradle the bottom of it as it expands up and out into the sky. Imagine that it keeps expanding, reaching out, and filling the entire universe. Extend your arms and palms up and out to the sides at a forty-five-degree angle (e).

Exhale and imagine the ball sinking in toward your tan tien. As the ball sinks and slightly contracts, let your body sink as well. Bend your knees slightly and lower your elbows toward your tan tien to accommodate the weight of the ball (f). Even when they contract, keep your palms and arms at a forty-five-degree angle up and out to the sides.

As you inhale, the ball lifts and expands out toward the universe again. Raise your body and arms to cradle and follow that expanding ball (g). Keep your arms at a forty-five-degree angle up and out to the sides. You can repeat this inhale-rise-expand, exhale-sink-contract cycle as many times as you like.

When it is time to bring this exercise to a close, let the ball sink down as you turn your palms downward and let them fall gradually to follow the sinking ball (h).

After the ball has sunk all the way down, allow it to shrink again, and put it back into your tan tien, bringing your hands back to their starting position (i). Meditate in this position for a while before coming out of the exercise. You can repeat this form again if you like or, better yet, flow right into the next exercise (Discharge Form).

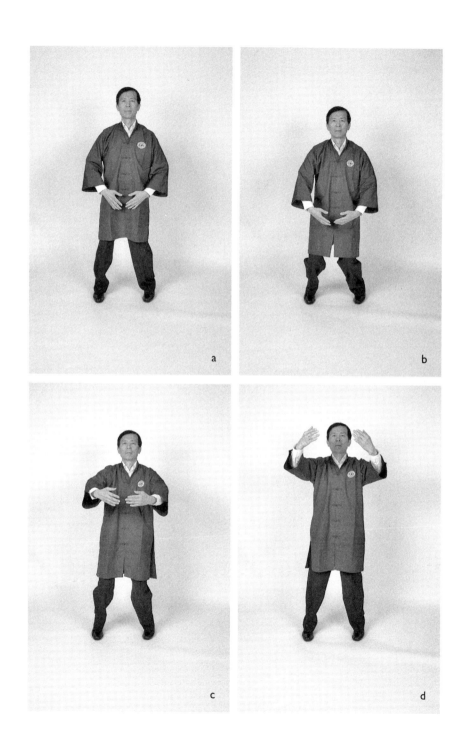

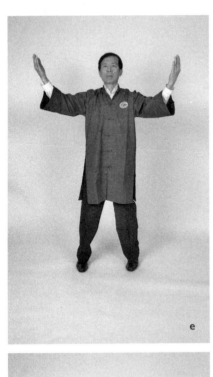

e

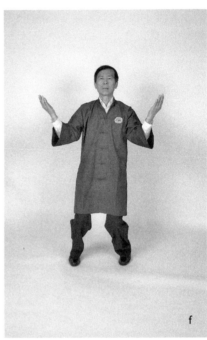

f

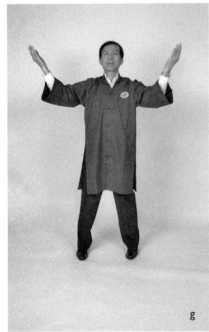

g

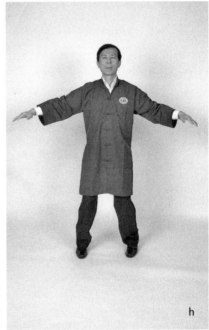

h

RESTORING YOUR LIFE ENERGY

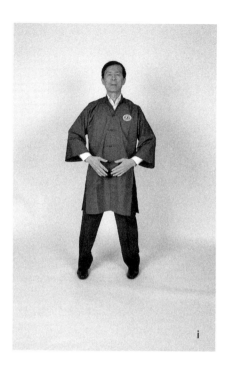

i

Benefits of Charge-Up Form

Why is it so important to do this exercise with a calm, pure mind in a location that is peaceful and pleasant? In Charge Up, we are opening up our energy, expanding that energy ball as a gesture to show that we wish to connect to the pure energy of the universe. To do this, we must be pure ourselves in this meditation.

We have to forget all the thoughts about what's going on in our own lives—the gossip at work, our family problems, last night's television show, and so on—and leave all those routine thoughts outside. We say to ourselves, "I just want to bring in pure universal energy." When we think about pure universal energy, we bring in pure universal energy. If we're thinking about bad energy or bad things, we can bring in a bad signal, a bad frequency or bad programming.

Energy comes to us like a key looking for a lock; one type of energy fits one type of lock. If you want to bring in pure universal energy, you must make yourself very pure and become a pure receptor. The type of energy you attract, the type that will cling to you, depends on what type of receptor you are. That's why it is important to do moving meditation with a calm mind. Put all your cares, nasty thoughts, and bad memories aside before you practice. Keep your mind pure and calm. If that is impossible, do something else for a while to calm down, then practice.

The reason we constantly let all the artificial bad energy from outside crash in on us and give us a hard time is because we don't use chi gung tools to clean ourselves and push it all back out. As soon as you radiate a clean message, the unclean or less powerful signal won't be able to cling to you. Each time you practice while you are feeling gentle, happy, easy, and relaxed, you take another step forward in cleaning up your energy. Your chi becomes clean, and your mind becomes pure.

Remember, in this form, you are using your ball of energy, imaginary or real, to touch the universe. This form reminds you why you learn how to move your energy to help your spiritual development. Ultimately, when you want to connect back to that pure One Energy of the Universe, can you use your physical hand to touch it? No. To connect with that energy, you need to use your energy. So you're not just reaching out with your hands and arms; you're reaching out with that imaginary ball of life energy.

This form is an important meditative gesture that imprints itself deep within us. It conveys our sense of humility, our need for nourishment and connection with our Source. It shows our sincerity and desire to become one with the Tao again. It is a wonderful way to reprogram our life energy with all these qualities.

Discharge Form

Negative energy is much heavier and vibrates at a lower frequency than clean, pure energy. In this moving meditation exercise, you are going to use the power of the earth's gravity—along with your calm, pure mind—to let go of your negative energy and let it drain away and return to the earth. The more calm and relaxed you are as you do this, the more effective it is.

Stand in tan tien meditation, as you center yourself and focus on that spot in the middle of your lower stomach (a). Calm your mind and prepare to let go of all the problems of the day, clear your thoughts, and focus on your breathing and the feeling in your lower abdomen.

Imagine an invisible ball expanding out from your tan tien, and allow your arms to follow that expanding ball, encircling it as it grows (b).

Let the ball keep expanding until it becomes very big. As it grows, it gets heavier and sinks down to the earth. Open and lower your arms, following that sinking ball. Imagine your tailbone pointing down toward the Earth; gently bend your knees (c). Stop your arms' expansion once they are at forty-five-degree angles down and out to the sides. Let go as the ball sinks.

As you exhale, allow your body to relax and sink. Focus on letting go of tension and cares. Keep your arms extended at forty-five-degree angles down and out to the sides (d). Imagine your fingertips pointing toward the earth; this helps guide that heavy energy by showing it where to go, allowing gravity to help pull it down and away. Keep your wrists softly bent and relaxed throughout this entire exercise. Relax and imagine letting go of any negativity or heaviness.

As you inhale, raise your body by thinking about the crown point at the top of your head. Let that point lift you up. At the same time, pull the tips of your elbows up, back, and in a little (e). Keep your wrists soft and your fingertips pointing down and out to the sides at forty-five-degree angles toward the ground during the entire movement of inhaling up and exhaling down.

Exhale and sink down through your tailbone, while you imagine it pointing down toward the earth; bend your knees (f). Again, let heavy, negative energy drain away down your arms and out through your fingertips into the earth. Repeat this inhalation and exhalation cycle in Discharge Form as many times as you like before coming back to end the exercise.

To close, gradually pull your elbows back and slowly bring your hands in front of your tan tien once again (g). You can repeat Discharge Form or, better yet, alternate it with a few repetitions of Charge-Up Form.

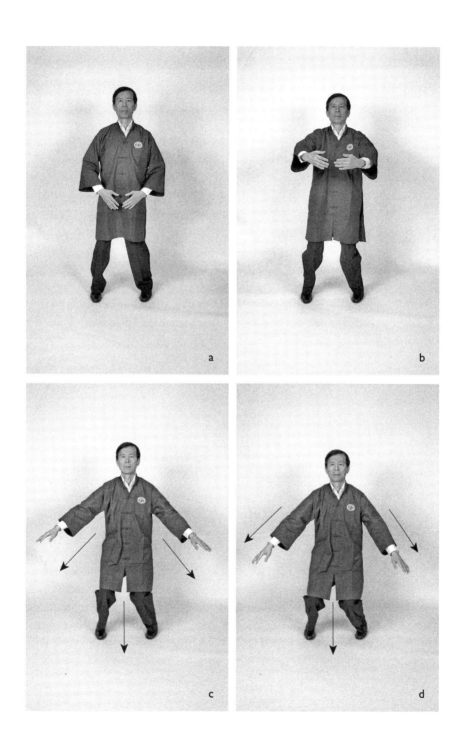

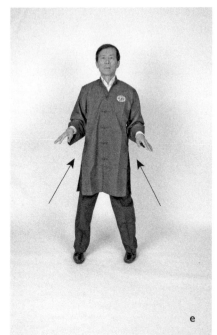

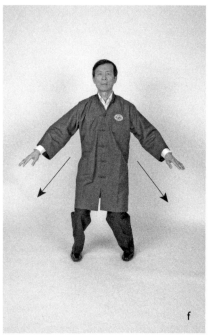

e

f

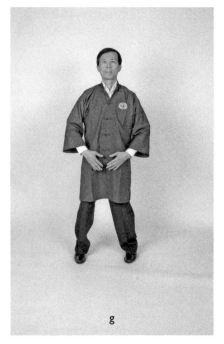

g

RESTORING YOUR LIFE ENERGY

Benefits of Discharge Form

The body is designed according to the natural laws of energy flow. Higher and lighter energy floats upward, while heavier, denser energy tends to sink. We take in nourishment or energy from the upper half of our body, and it flows downward during digestion so that we may release waste products through the lower part of our body into the earth.

Likewise when we practice chi gung, we open ourselves up to receive and connect to lighter, higher-frequency energy by letting our energy ball rise up and out (Charge-Up Form). We release used, heavy, unwanted energy by expanding that ball downward while we relax our entire body and let go (Discharge Form).

Alternating the Charge-Up and Discharge Forms is a good way to pump the internal energy circulation within your body. Alternating the two forms pulls new, fresh energy in, while pushing old, heavy energy out.

Even though you are letting go of and draining away negative energy in Discharge Form, you will still have much better results if you do it when you are calm and relaxed. Resist practicing the form when you are upset or in a disruptive location. Whenever you use moving meditation, even when you practice discharging negative energy, you are bringing your mind and chi together to connect and communicate with each other. You don't want to connect with your life energy with an upset, fearful, or angry mind and risk contaminating or reinforcing that bad programming to your chi. Instead, you want to reprogram it with that message of letting go.

When you practice Discharge Form, you may be working with just your imagination at first. However, the more you practice, the more you may start to sense something draining from your fingertips or feel a connection between your fingertips and the earth. This is normal. Don't focus on it too much. Continue to relax and let go!

Compress T'ai Chi Ball

T'ai chi ball is another name for that imaginary energy ball you have been working with. Remember that *t'ai chi* simply means the ultimate state of chi.

This exercise is also used in Tao gung, or "Tao's work," meditation practice. It is a very advanced meditative form designed to purify your life energy. It can also refine that energy into a higher-frequency signal we call *jing*. Jing will supercharge your life energy signal and is often used by advanced practitioners in the healing and martial arts applications of t'ai chi.

The focus of this meditation is in front of the heart, a location governed by an energy center known as the *middle tan tien*. It is a very important exercise for anyone struggling with a health problem.

Stand in the same tan tien meditation that serves as the beginning to all moving meditation forms (a). Remain here as long as you like, until you feel calm and centered and ready to begin.

Allow a ball of energy to expand outward in front of you from your tan tien. Move your palms to hold the imaginary ball and follow it as it gets bigger (b).

Imagine the invisible ball of energy getting bigger and bigger, sinking and expanding toward infinity downward through the earth, as far as the edge of the universe underneath you. As it expands downward, imagine gathering all the energy in the universe below you.

Now think of the imaginary ball growing even bigger and expanding to the edge of the universe behind you. As it expands backward to infinity, let it push your arms behind you slightly as you work to gather in all the energy in the universe behind you (c).

As the imaginary ball keeps expanding, imagine you are gathering all the energy of the universe from the edge of infinity to your right and left sides; bring your arms up and around from behind (d). You should look like you are about to give someone a big hug.

Now that you've gathered the entire universe from below, behind, and both sides of you, begin to hug your arms around that huge imaginary ball of energy in front of your chest (e). As you are hugging, grab all the energy of the universe from in front of you as well. Imagine you are reaching all the way out to the edge of infinity, gathering in all that energy so that you can add it to your imaginary ball.

Now imagine you are embracing the whole universe inside that ball in front of your chest. Keeping your arms at shoulder-height and your fingertips pointing toward each other, bring your arms together in front of you (f). Don't let your fingertips touch.

Gradually let your elbows sink and your fingertips to begin pointing upward (g). As they do, imagine pulling all the remaining energy from the universe above you into that ball you are holding in front of your chest. As your elbows sink and your fingertips point up, your imaginary ball holding the entire universe slowly shrinks to fit inside the space between your palms.

Now imagine that the ball is condensing and compressing, getting smaller and smaller between your palms. You are compressing and condensing the whole universe in all directions into a tiny ball between your palms in front of your heart. Point your fingertips upward. Do not touch your palms together; keep them slightly apart to make room for that energy ball you are compressing (h).

Your imaginary ball can be as big as a baseball or small like a ping-pong ball. If you are very focused and practice a long time, you can make it even smaller, like the size of a marble or a pea. Stay with whatever size ball can firmly hold your feeling, concentration, and imagination between the center points of your palms.

Don't let the sides of your hands touch your body. Keep them slightly away from but in front of the middle of your chest as you hold and compress that imaginary ball. Your energy ball is now lined up with your middle tan tien, the energy center in the middle of your chest, near your heart (i).

Meditate in this position, focusing on your ball. Beam the center of each palm into the center of the ball. Close your eyes and look into it. Send your sense of smell, taste, and feeling into it. If your mind wanders, bring it back to think about that tiny energy ball you are holding between your palms. As you inhale, the energy ball tries to expand and may push your palms apart ever so slightly.

As you exhale, the ball compresses again, and your relaxed palms gently move or push closer together without touching. Inhale and exhale, expand and compress, holding that ball in front of your chest with your full concentration. Imagine you are holding and compressing the entire universe. Don't be surprised if you start to feel some sensation between your palms.

Meditate in this manner for as long as you are comfortable.

After a while, allow the center of that ball to beam straight up like a laser through the space between your palms. As it does, imagine the ball starting to rise, and follow it with your palms (j). Let the ball travel upward, parallel to and along the centerline of your body—in front of your nose, between your eyebrows, and directly parallel to your crown point.

As the imaginary energy ball keeps beaming and traveling upward, follow it with your palms. Imagine the ball traveling through the universe as high as it can go, trying to reach infinity. Follow with your arms, keeping them very relaxed, until they reach a point where they can no longer rise comfortably (k). Don't raise them so high that you stiffen or hyperextend your arms. Hold them up but slightly relaxed. Keep your feet flat on the floor; no need to stand on your toes.

Once your imaginary ball has gone as high as it can, feel it begin to expand. It starts to open up from the upper edge of the universe, growing wider in all directions and following the edges of the universe as it expands. Let the energy open and fill the entire universe once again. As it expands, allow the ball to open your arms as well so they follow its expansion. Your arms open and start to lower as if they are tracing the outline of a giant circle (l).

Feel the ball continue to open like a blossom, filling the entire universe. Bring your hands and arms down and reach out as they open, tracing the edges of the universe (m).

Now that the energy ball has completed its expansion, filling all directions of the universe once again, bring your hands and arms to rest, still holding that ball, at a forty-five-degree angles down and out to the side from your tan tien (n). You can meditate here for a little while, inhaling and exhaling, as you gently expand and contract your entire body with your breathing. You can even pretend you can still feel the gentle expanding and contracting of the imaginary ball of universal energy, following along with your inhalation and exhalation.

When you are finished, gather all that energy of the universe back into a ball, and return the ball of energy back to your tan tien (o). Stay in tan tien meditation for as long as you wish, or do more repetitions of Compress T'ai Chi Ball.

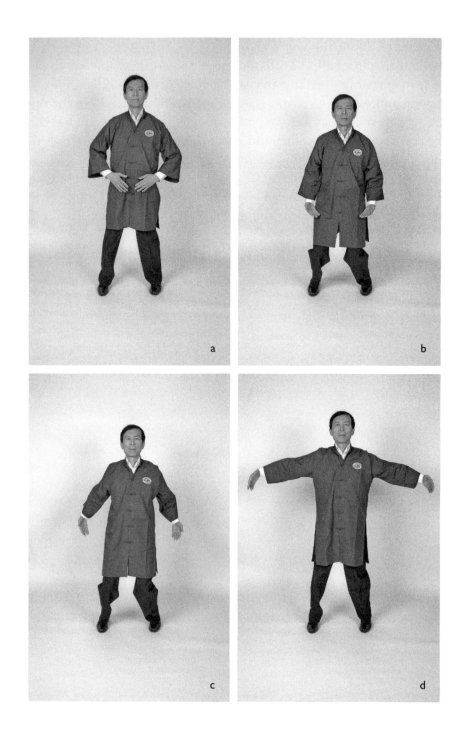

a

b

c

d

RESTORING YOUR LIFE ENERGY

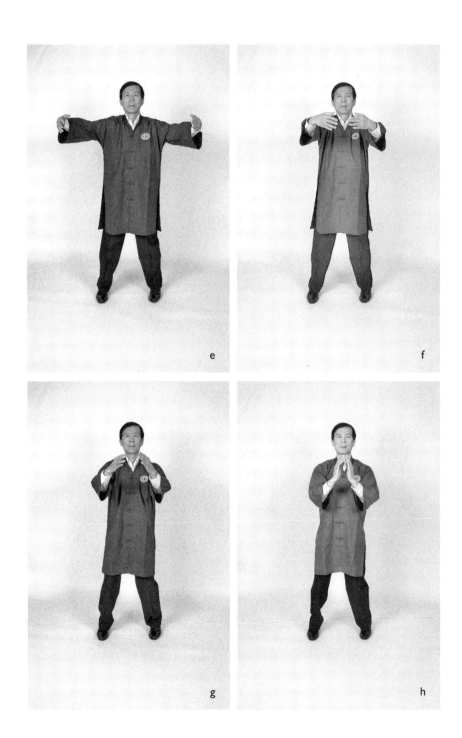

e

f

g

h

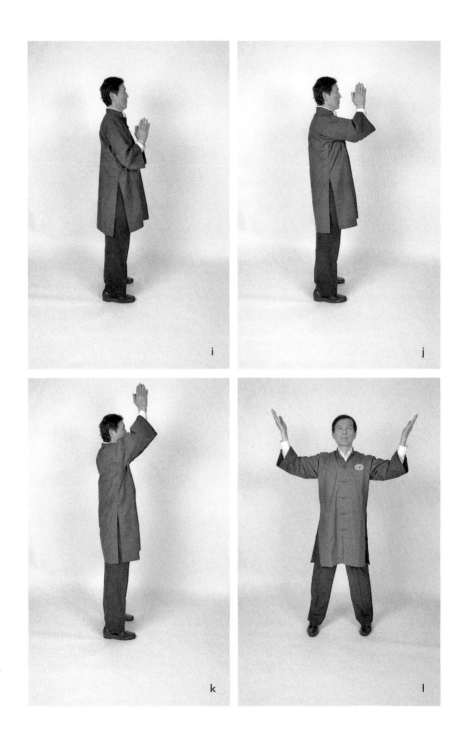

RESTORING YOUR LIFE ENERGY

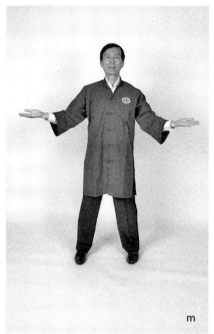

m

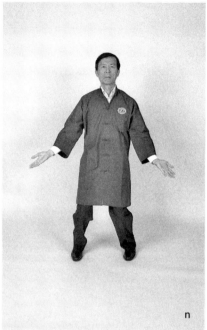

n

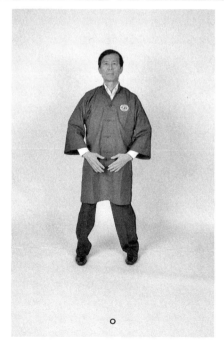

o

Benefits of Compress T'ai Chi Ball

The center of our life energy resides in our lower tan tien, which is located behind the navel in the lower stomach. That's why all of our moving meditation exercises begin and end there. However, there are two other major energy centers in our body: the middle tan tien, which is in the center of our chest, near the heart; and the upper tan tien, which is in the center of our head, directly behind the spot in the middle of our eyebrows.

Although the lower tan tien is the root or origin of our life energy, it is the middle tan tien that governs health issues. Just look at how many critical life functions are regulated in the upper torso area. Since the middle tan tien governs several main functions that are key to our well-being and health, when we want to work on healing, we go to the middle tan tien.

The upper tan tien energy center in our head makes possible the thinking and sensory perceptions we enjoy. In moving meditation, we leave this energy center alone. We don't go to there until we are pure, because our head has a tendency to be misguided by our sensory perceptions, outside input, and artificial thinking. This is also why meditations that focus on the head or points inside it can lead to more risks of illusions, hallucinations, or mental disturbances if we are not careful. Many schools focus on a specific point in the center of the head to meditate. When advanced t'ai chi and Tao gung practitioners focus on the upper tan tien point, it is so they can ultimately move it, bringing it down to connect with the lower tan tien, so their mind can return to its root.

Our Compress T'ai Chi Ball meditation starts from the lower tan tien as we first expand that ball outward. Eventually, it comes together and focuses in front of the middle tan tien. Later, it passes in front of and through the upper tan tien before rejoining the energy of the universe. Then we carefully bring all that energy back into the lower tan tien again. In our practice, that original center of life energy in the lower tan tien is always the beginning and the end—it is always the boss.

While we compress the entire universe into a small ball between our palms, that tremendous force of concentration and compression becomes like a refiner's oven. It burns, purifies, and refines our energy. The more we can focus our senses, thinking, and feeling, into that little ball, the hotter the oven gets.

When you first start this practice, you may feel like you are holding something the size of a baseball in front of your chest. Over time, see if you can make that ball even smaller, perhaps to the size of a ping-pong ball, then a marble, then a pea, then a pellet. The smaller your ball, the more intense your focus and the hotter your oven. This type of concentration burns away a lot of pollution from your energy, just like fire refines steel. When your focus is really sincere and concentrated, only pure mind and pure life energy can fit inside the ball. It is so small, so condensed, that anything else that wants to sneak inside it cannot fit.

8

CONCLUSION

EACH OF US is uniquely made of universal energy in the form of life energy, or chi. We do not own life energy; it is owned by the Tao. But we depend on it to function in this dimension, our present world.

This life energy force has its own agenda. It is programmed to propel forward through birth, growth, and reproduction in its own natural way. It has its own set of requirements to thrive. Any condition contrary to this natural state of chi will reduce its full function and performance. That's why we experience aging, illness, and death. So our goal—indeed, our duty—is to find a way to reduce those conditions contrary to the inherent nature of life energy and instead learn to cooperate with and allow our chi to thrive in its natural state of harmony.

True chi gung, or chi's work, is designed to restore and cooperate with the natural way of chi, not force it to fit into our own agenda. We can only work with chi by following the natural laws and inclination of its original program. We cannot force it to change its nature. However, we can make it strong again by restoring our life energy to its natural state. We accomplish this, not by tricks or force, but by yielding to its nature. Only in this way will our chi again flow easily and regain the strength of its original signal.

The concept of yielding is key. In all chi gung exercises, we are constantly working toward the ability to actually feel our life energy, so we can ultimately learn to yield, cooperate, and flow with it. Through calm concentration on the feeling of this energy, we allow our chi to return back to its original state, the state we experienced as unborn babies. When we yield to such pure, clean chi, it sends back a strong signal that provides healing and nurturing to our physical body.

Chi's signal is, by nature, weak and delicate. You cannot feel that force in your body that is currently at work dividing your cells, pulling in nourishment through cellular membranes, or activating your immune system's defenses. Even though these forces are so subtle and "weak," you could not live without them. This subtlety, this barely perceptible weakness, is why we must, in turn, become very calm, quiet, sincere, and yielding in order to feel and work with life energy.

As soon as you feel any sensation of chi, stay, follow, and work with it with a soft and slow motion. Yield and stay with your chi. Don't push it, but don't forget about or detach from it either. It's a delicate balance of feeling and flowing that can take a while to learn.

Lao Tzu talks quite often in the *Tao Te Ching* about the power of gentleness and yielding:

> When people are born, they are gentle and weak.
> At death they are hard and stiff.
> Green plants are pliant and tender while living.
> When they're dead, they are withered and dried.
> Therefore the stiff and unbending follow death.
> The supple and yielding follow life.[1]

Suppleness and yielding are not only important in terms of our body when we practice, they are important states of mind. To reach this delicate balance of being able to feel and work with chi, we must throw out our ego and selfishness when we practice. We cannot rush this. We cannot enter a pure state with the "stiffness" of a desire to achieve some result. Neither can we give up. We have to remain on the fine dividing line between "not too much and not too little," as the ancient chi masters advised.

RESTORING YOUR LIFE ENERGY

Once we feel a sensation of our chi in one area of our body, we work slowly to expand this feeling to the entire body. *Work* means that we let the chi reach out to every part of our body; we don't try to force it to do so.

You see, chi only works by flow, not by jumping. We cannot force our chi to move from point A to point B; rather, we must flow continuously from point to point, like a line connecting a series of dots. An even better analogy would be flow our chi like water seeping through a paper towel.

It takes time to develop chi's work and to restore chi's original state. Do not rush for results. Live with it every day, every hour, every minute. Try to feel life energy all the time, like an unborn baby. An unborn baby doesn't take time out to feel and yield to its life energy; such work is its natural state of being.

If you embrace them, every concept and practice in this book can help you restore your life energy. These practices and teachings, passed down through the centuries of Taoist wisdom, are very valuable—even priceless. You may say, "Master, I happen to have a couple thousand dollars. Can I buy some chi from you?" Save your couple thousand dollars. Go home and feel it. We get used to thinking that whenever we need something, we can go and buy it. Restored chi is something you cannot buy. Likewise, the life energy we are talking about is not theory or philosophy or an idea that we invented. It's real, palpable, and you can learn to feel it.

Don't worry or berate yourself if you cannot feel anything for a while. Everyone's experience of chi feeling depends on their physical and energy states. If you have an injury or illness, you might feel your chi later on in your practice, after a few weeks or months. Another person who is young and healthy may feel differently or sooner. The way people describe their feeling of chi varies, not only from person to person, but from week to week, month to month, and year to year. During the process of training, the feeling changes and improves. So don't pay too much attention to any one sensation or give up due to a lack of sensation at first. Everybody is different. As long as you are putting in a sincere effort to practice in the right way and are heading in the right direction, your practice will bear fruit sooner or later.

Having a master who really knows about chi and how to strengthen and repair it helps a lot. But there are so few left today who carry the old Taoist wisdom on life energy. That ancient temple lifestyle and its monks have mostly disappeared. I count myself lucky to have grabbed the tail end of that era as a young teenager, and I teach others in order to preserve what was passed down to me. The core of that knowledge is that each of us has this boundless miracle called life energy inside us, and through that miracle, we have a chance to reconnect to the Tao.

In this book, we've delved inward to explore the energy within that tiny first cell. We've also expanded our energy outward to enfold the entire universe. That, too, is the heart of this wisdom: the piece of original life energy inside you is both infinitely small and infinitely large. When you can connect to that unlimited power, you will rediscover your True Self and reach your true potential.

NOTES

CHAPTER 2. How Chi Gets Damaged, Weakened, or Blocked

1. *Tao Te Ching,* Chapters 10, 20, 52, 64, and 81.

CHAPTER 3. Restoring the Life Energy Signal

1. *Tao Te Ching,* Chapter 42.
2. *Tao Te Ching,* Chapter 48.

CHAPTER 4. Making the Chi Connection for Health

1. *Tao Te Ching,* Chapter 25.

CHAPTER 6. Moving Meditation: The Key

1. *Tao Te Ching,* Chapter 55.

CHAPTER 7. Cleaning and Restoring Your Life Energy

1. *Tao Te Ching,* Chapter 14.
2. *Tao Te Ching,* Chapter 12.

CHAPTER 8. Conclusion

6. *Tao Te Ching,* Chapter 76.

BOOKS BY MASTER WAYSUN LIAO

Chi: Discovering Your Life Energy

Chi is the invisible energy of life that flows in and around us throughout the universe. Used skillfully, it can have a remarkable effect on health and vitality—to the degree that you'd be tempted to call it magical, if it weren't so completely natural. Here is a perfect introduction to chi that explains in a direct and simple way what it is and why it is essential to a healthy and vital life. It provides an easy-to-understand explanation of chi, and then helps readers recognize, develop, and strengthen their own chi through specific breathing techniques and basic exercises, all demonstrated by the author.

The Essence of T'ai Chi

The deepest benefits of T'ai Chi cannot be realized without an understanding of its underlying principles. This book presents these principles through translations of three core classics of T'ai Chi that are often considered the "T'ai Chi Bible," accompanied by the author's insightful commentary. Master Liao demonstrates how to increase the body's inner energy (*chi*) and transform it into power, health, and well-being. By reading the clear and precise explanations of the fundamental principles of T'ai Chi, students can develop a more complete understanding of the art and philosophy of this traditional martial art.

T'ai Chi Classics

According to Master Liao, the great power of T'ai Chi cannot be realized without knowing its inner meaning. *T'ai Chi Classics* presents the inner meaning and techniques of T'ai Chi movements through translations of three core classics of T'ai Chi. The texts are introduced by three chapters explaining how to increase inner energy (*chi*), transform it into inner power (*jing*), and project this inner power outward to repel an opponent without physical contact. Master Liao also provides a description of the entire sequence of T'ai Chi movements, illustrated by his own line drawings.

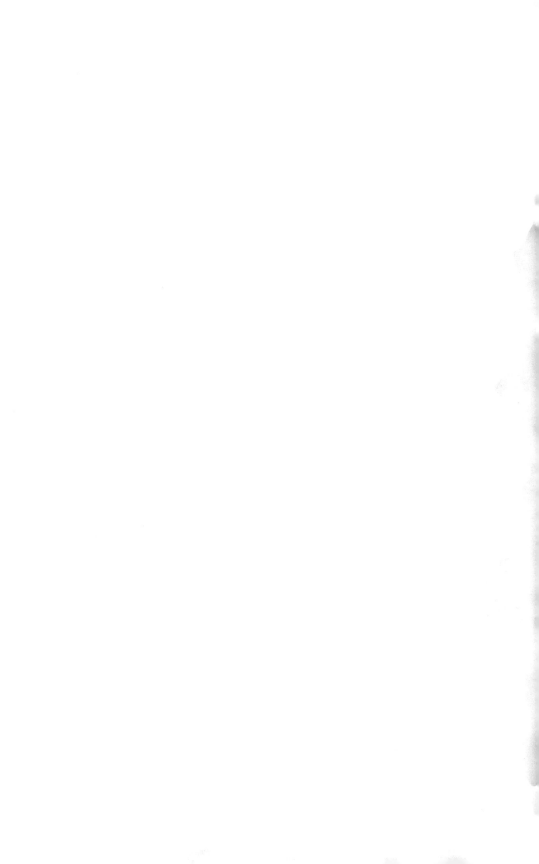